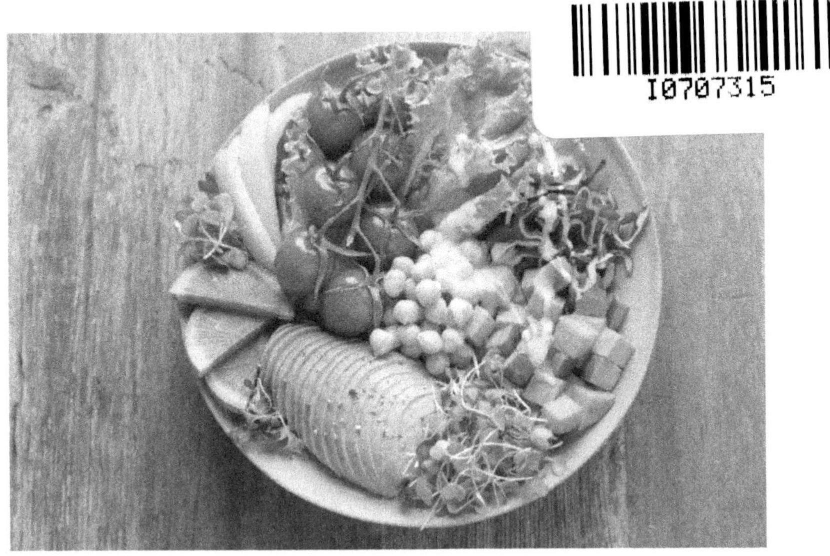

Plant Based Diet
for Beginners

Plant Based Diet Meal Plan, Plant Based Cookbook, with Easy, Delicious and Healthy Whole Food Recipes

By Silvia Pala

mentioned or alluded to in this book. The information presented is purely for your benefit and not ours, in any way, and does not imply that the author or publisher endorses or is affiliated with the individual, organization, website, product or company mentioned herein. Readers should be aware that any websites or online materials referenced may not be available after the publication of this book, because the author and publisher do not take any liability for maintaining third party or external sources referenced.

Table of Contents

[Foreword] It's Not What We Eat, But How and When

I was overjoyed when Silvia asked me to write a foreword for this book. I've been through pretty much every aspect of every diet… I grew up hunting and fishing with my father in Northern Minnesota. Then, due to high cholesterol levels and fear of a heart attack (which is in my genetic family history), I became a vegetarian. I've since done week-long fasts, dabbled in raw food, and have studied 'proper food combining' extensively. I've been in tantra yoga sessions that are hours long, holding poses for more than 15 minutes while our teacher expounds upon the negative ramifications (spiritually) of garlic.

My grandmother and great-grandmother both owned restaurants, and the former published her own cookbook twice. I guess a love of food runs in my veins!

It's amazing to me that know what's in food – the nutrients, calories, vitamins, minerals – but don't really know how to best absorb those throughout our digestive tract. I see it often in my patients I treat with Bioresonance: Malnutrition, malabsorption, mineral and/or fatty acid deficiency… all those lead to serious health consequences many years down the road. My colleague Carol Miller, a certified Nutritional Therapist, also sees the same problems in the large majority of her clients.

I dare say that there are only two reasons we grow old: lack of absorbing life (life-giving nutrients and raw experiences life has to offer) and a negative mindset.

That's why I congratulate you, the reader, for picking up this book! It's more than just a collection of recipes; Silvia has lovingly and painstakingly gathered a broad array of recipes to suit a number of healthy diets – including properly combined ones – and has also included the nutritional information for each. Being healthy, feeling young, and always bringing your best game doesn't happen by taking a miracle supplement once a day. It's a journey of a thousand steps… you start by making small changes to how you cook, being conscious of small choices you make, and then all of a sudden you'll wake up one day and notice that the pain in your lower back is gone, for example, or that you recover much faster from a workout or that you no longer experience hangovers. Living a healthy life isn't a 'diet', it's the way you live your life.

And that's why we should put a modern spin on the centuries-old adage "you are what you eat" – because you're so much more than that. It's no longer two-dimensional. You aren't just *what* you eat, but also *when* and *how*.

Have fun reading this book, and may you live happy, healthy, and always smiling!

Kasey Phifer
Bristol, England

[Introduction] A Love for Food, Generations Deep

Modern day Italian cuisine is known and loved the world over – food is simply in my genes. I grew up watching my grandparents cooking and singing happily in the kitchen. Later, I would help them during shopping trips to the markets and the store, learning how to determine the freshness of produce by pressing with my finger along the edges or tips, pulling a pineapple leaf out of the center easily, and other little tricks that one simply learns during practice.

I've written this book as a way to help you dive into the world of food from the absolute beginning. I explain how to cut and prepare vegetables, how to compile a shopping list, and make a balanced meal plan for the week.

Given that I've included all the helpful details you'd need for a recipe: The time it takes to prepare and cook, vegan / proper food combining substitutes, and nutritional information. If I've left anything out, **please let me know in the reviews on Amazon**. I'll update those areas in the second edition.

What was your motivation for selecting this book? Please let me know your feedback and thoughts by **leaving a review on Amazon**, *because this 'open' way of communicating may help others who have read the book or are interested in reading it. You can always contact me by email (mentioned at the beginning of this book) if you're not comfortable* **leaving a review on Amazon**.

A Brief Summary of What's Ahead

Here's what you can expect in this book:

- A short description of various diets, plant-based diets, and even those that incorporate some meat.
- List of ailments and diseases that a plant-based diet can alleviate
- Healthy foods, foods to avoid, and helpful information about them
- Recipes for every meal and snack
- Meal plans complete with grocery shopping lists

- Shopping tips
- Storage tips to eliminate food waste
- What to expect and prepare for when switching to a plant-based diet
- Helpful resources & references for further reading
- Helpful quick guides, such as measurement conversions to metric, rules for proper food combining, and other information you might like to look up quickly

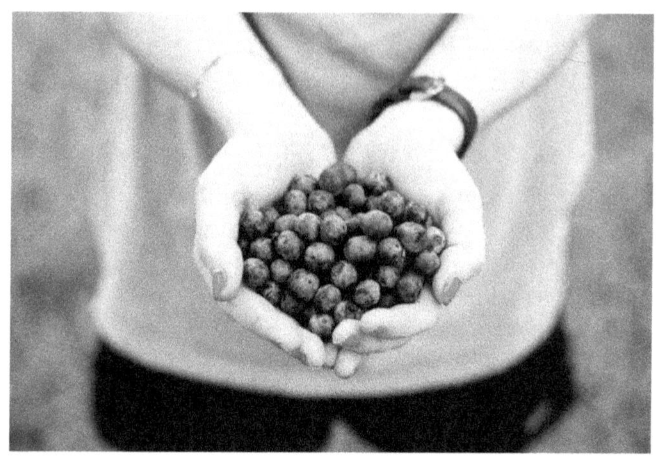

[1] What A Plant-Based Diet Is and Entails

A plant-based diet is one consisting entirely or in large part of foods derived from plants, including vegetables, legumes, grains, fruits, seeds, and nuts. Animal-based or animal-derived products are usually seldom found in plant-based diets. If someone does not eat animal products at all, they are considered vegan – and we'll delve more into that subject in sub-chapter 1.2. below.

[1.1] Origins of Plant-Based Diets

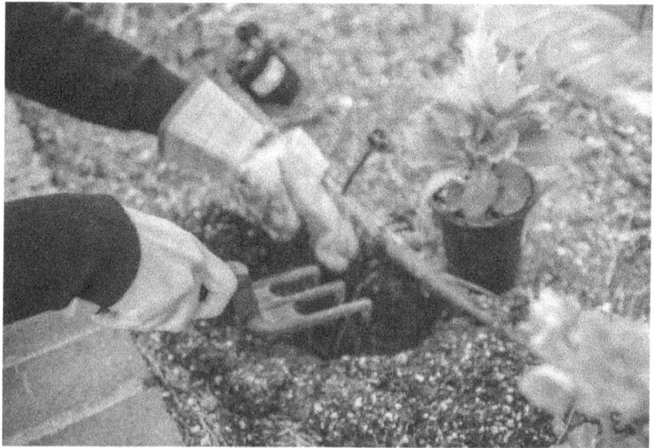

The exact origins of plant-based diets are unknown. It is assumed that when we were hunter gatherers thousands of years ago, we lived largely from plants, roots, seeds, flowers, nuts, fruits and vegetables. Eating meat was a very rare occasion, often consumed once a month or less.

As humans became agrarians, and relied more upon raising crops and livestock for their food, they started eating more and more foods that were high in protein but harmful to the gut: Cow milk, sheep's milk, eggs, meat, shellfish, and fish all have high protein content, but all have enzymes that get stuck in our intestinal lining, thereby blocking the absorption of nutrients and creating inflammation.

It has only been the past hundred years or so that humans have 'rediscovered' purely plant-based diets for their health benefits. One of the most notable vegetarians was, in fact, Adolf Hitler! Leonardo da Vinci and Gandhi were also vegetarians.

[1.2] Types of (Plant-Based) Diets

Here are all diet types that are more well-known or popular currently:

1. **Vegetarian** – do not eat meat, poultry (chicken, fowl, birds) or fish. They do eat cheese, milk, and dairy commonly, because the general rule of thumb is that an animal hasn't died in order for a vegetarian to eat.

2. **Pescatarian** – A vegetarian who eats fish, but no meat or poultry. They often also consume eggs and dairy, but this isn't included in the definition.

3. **Vegan** – Does not eat any products from animals, excluding butter, milk, honey, leather products worn like shoes / jackets / handbags, and does not use cosmetics that have been tested on animals. Even some medications and pills are made with lactose or milk derivatives, so vegans must read ingredient labels carefully.

4. **Fruitarian** – they take it one step further than vegans, eating only the 'fruit' of plants. This is based on the premise that even life on different levels of consciousness is sacred, and so only the fruit – which is essentially discarded from a plant or tree – can be consumed without causing harm or 'killing'

any plants, trees, grains, or other living flora in our environment.

5. **Ketogenic** – the 'keto' diet is high in fat, allows a moderate amount of protein, and heavily restricts the intake of carbohydrates, even from fruits and vegetables. This transitions the body into a ketogenic state, one where it burns fats for energy rather than carbs or sugars.

6. **Atkins** – the Atkins diet was very popular about one decade ago. It's nearly identical to a keto diet, except that it is high in protein and fat, and very low in carbohydrates.

7. **Paleolithic** – a 'Paleo' diet for short reasons that we humans should eat as we allegedly did many centuries ago, approximately after fire was invented but before we settled down and learned how to sow oats, grains, and barley. Similar to 'proper food combining', they alter their food in a way as to make it more readily digestible. (More on this subject later.)

8. **Proper food combining** – this niche diet gained considerable traction in the 1980s and still continues to be celebrated by food nutritionists and natural health specialists. The goal is to eat only certain foods combined together so that our digestive tract absorbs the maximum amount of nutrients from our meal.

Later in this chapter I'll go into detail on a few of the above diets, because they warrant more detail and explanation as to the science and reasoning behind their 'rules'.

[1.3] Overview of Health Benefits of Plant-Based Diets

There are literally entire books written on the health benefits of plant-based diets, and how they have reversed or cured many diseases. I don't delve into much detail on those subjects individually in this book, because I wanted to keep the focus on how you can use these diets in real life, and with practical takeaways to make your life easier.

Here are some movies and documentaries that will inspire you during the rough moments of your newly adopted vegan or veggie pledge, or help persuade those you love who have questions about your lifestyle change:

- Food Inc. (2008) – documentary by Robert Kenner analyzing our food chain and restaurants being dominated by large corporations
- Forks Over Knives (2011) – documentary by Lee Fulkerson and John Corry that looks deeply at the very real possibility of eliminating and/or controlling diseases such as cancer and diabetes by switching to a plant-based diet
- Super Size Me (2004) – documentary by Morgan Spurlock where he attempts to live one month entirely off McDonald's food and suffers severe health consequences; there is also a sequel, "Super Size Me 2"
- Veducated (2011) – documentary chronicling the challenges of three New Yorkers who love meat and dairy as they adopt a 6-week long vegan diet
- The Invisible Vegan (2019) – documenting the shift toward conscious eating and behaviour in America

Books that I've consulted and that you'll also find inspiring have been included at the end of this book in Appendix D: Resources.

Prevention, Management & Reversal

Altering your diet has been linked in thousands of studies across the globe to positive effects and outcomes on one's health. A few of these commonly occurring diseases will be covered in more detail in chapter three.

Just to spark your curiosity, some of the diseases that can be prevented, managed (that is, the worsening of it has been halted), recovered from faster, and reversed or 'cured' as stated in The Encyclopedia of Natural Medicine by Murray and Pizzorno, N.D.s (more in Appendix D) is in brief here:

- AIDS & HIV
- Alcoholism
- Allergies
- Asthma

- Alzheimer's
- ADD
- Bipolar
- Cancer
- Chronic Candidiasis
- Carpal Tunnel Syndrome
- Cataracts
- High Cholesterol
- Chronic Fatigue Syndrome
- Depression
- Diabetes Mellitus
- Eczema
- Fibrocystic Breast Disease
- Fibromyalgia
- Food Allergies
- Gout
- Heart Disease
- Hepatitis
- Herpes
- Inflammatory Bowel Disease
- Insomnia
- Irritable Bowel Syndrome
- Kidney Stones
- Osteoarthritis
- Premenstrual Syndrome
- Prostate Enlargement
- Psoriasis
- Rheumatoid Arthritis
- Seasonal Affective Disorder
- Bacterial Sinusitis
- Ulcers (Duodenal and Gastric)
- Vaginitis
- Varicose Veins

[1.4] Possible Health Risks & Adverse Consequences

In the many studies available on the Internet, at the library, and in university libraries, I found little to no adverse health effects due to eating a plant-based diet. There are only two staple nutrients that should be watched out for if a person is not consuming animal products:

B12: This vitamin helps red blood cells divide naturally, same as Folic Acid or Folate (known as B9). This is only naturally found in animal foods, but not in honey. B12 is in meat, poultry, and fish and humans consuming those substances (or "foods" if you will) can readily access and assimilate that B12. The plant-based B12 cannot be assimilated by our human digestive tract, because it must first be broken down by bacteria.

But that's good news! B12 can be 'prepared' for our consumption by bacteria, not involving any harm to animals. Look for foods fortified with B12 such as cereals, grains, breads, and juices. Or, take a supplement of B12.

On a personal note, I know of two women who have carried out their pregnancy from conception to parturition while being on a completely vegan diet. They each had two children who are being raised vegan. They take daily supplements, and are healthy, happy, and beautiful children! It might have been the case back in 1955 when the link between veganism and lack of B12 (and corresponding / resulting damage to nerves) was first established – but we haven't had to worry about those possible negative consequences for decades if we simply inform ourselves before making a decision.

Iron: This mineral's main duty is to carry oxygen throughout the body in red blood cells, and also help remove carbon dioxide. If your iron levels are low, you'll feel tired or fatigued, sometimes dizzy, and your blood will have a difficult time clotting or coagulating, which is necessary to stop bleeding. Iron can be found naturally in plant forms, but this 'non-hemme' type, as it's called, isn't as readily absorbed by humans as the hemme type of iron found in animal meat.

It's best to consume iron with Vitamin C, to help your body absorb it better. Drinking caffeine doesn't necessarily lower your iron levels as such -- as the old wives' tale warns us. Caffeine damages Vitamin C in our stomachs and upper digestional tract, thereby hindering our absorption of iron. Plant sources that are high in iron include: lentils, garbanzo beans / chickpeas, tofu, cashews, spinach, pumpkin seeds, and kale -- just to name a few.

[1.5] Plant-Based vs. Other (Meat) Diets

There are many types of diets and lifestyle habits out there. This subchapter briefly explains all the more common and popular ones, so you can decide which feels right for you and inform yourself more about these using some of the resources in Appendix D: References.

Ketogenic

This is a high-fat, low-carb diet recommending adequate amounts of protein. It's been recommended to prevent epilepsy outbursts in children, as well as to promote weight loss. The body, by consuming high amounts of fat but low or no carbohydrates, then burns fat for energy. Ketones can be measured in the urine to find out the body's level of ketosis, or how well it's converting fat into energy to burn -- rather than carbohydrates.

Atkins

The Atkins diet was very popular in the 1990s and early 2000s in the USA. Similar to a ketogenic diet, it promotes high fat and low carbohydrate intake, but it differs from the keto diet in two important ways: (1) It promotes high intake of proteins rather than moderate / adequate amounts. (2) Foods with high glycemic indexes such as white bread and refined sugar are 'banned' from the diet as well as foods with low glycemic indexes like wild rice and certain vegetables. Because different carbohydrates have a different effect on our body's ability to produce insulin, ignoring this difference proved to cause cravings and binges is the followers of the diet. Other sources state that it created a high risk of heart disease.

Paleo

A 'paleolithic' diet is similar to Keto and Atkins at first glance. It promotes low consumption of carbohydrates in what we would consider the 'classic' form, such as bread or rice.

Paleo diets are based on the premise that our guts haven't evolved as quickly as our modern technology and behaviour. Hence why eating similar to what paleolithic people have eaten might be good for the body. It also looks at macro nutrients and our body's ability to digest nutrition present in the food we consume.

Many people think that a paleo diet is simply gluten-free, or raw. This isn't 100% the case. Many studies (listed in the 'further reading' section in the appendix) point to serious health conditions arising from the consumption of gluten, such as gut inflammation, malabsorption of nutrients, skin problems, mental health issues, and autoimmune diseases. Even grains and legumes that do not contain gluten are avoided because they contain phytic acid and lectins which can prevent the absorption of some minerals into the bloodstream or damage the gut lining, which impairs absorption of nutrients. (See "Eat Drink Paleo" in the appendix.)

In a sense, nature has planned things in a very smart way. Seeds are high in enzyme inhibitors which prevent them from sprouting early. If a plant started growing in the dead of winter, it wouldn't have much chance of survival. So when spring comes around and soaks the ground in water, the water removes those enzyme inhibitors, leaving the nutrients to which they were bound.

Grains to avoid on a Paleo diet:
- wheat
- barley
- rye
- corn / maize
- spelt
- bran
- millet
- oats

- brown / white / wild rice

Legumes must be fermented, sprouted or soaked so that they are 'safe' to eat. Soy products such as tofu, soymilk and meat substitutes are the most harmful to our gut, according to leading Paleo experts. Miso (fermented tofu) a naturally brewed wheat and gluten-free soy sauce can be consumed occasionally. Legumes to avoid on a Paleo diet:

- soy beans
- black-eyed / pinto beans
- red kidney beans
- cannellini beans
- dried or split peas
- lentils
- chickpeas / garbanzo beans
- butter beans

Notice how potatoes, sweet potatoes, yams, and winter squash are not in the list above. Due to space (and reader's comments / suggestions), I'm only briefly touching on each diet and what they entail. If your interest is aroused or it sounds like it's for you, then you can look up more information on the subject from other resources. The tubers I mentioned at the beginning of this paragraph are considerably high in carbohydrate content (more than 20 grams of carbs per 100 grams of product). They are recommended in moderation because the idea is to have the body take energy from vegetables, animal products, and meat. Potatoes and the like should be soaked (and some recommend peeling them) to remove the enzyme inhibitors from their peels which do damage to the gut.

"Pseudograins" have anti-nutrient properties similar to grains and legumes. But because they typically have more protein, B vitamins, healthy fatty acids and iron, they're considered 'safer' to eat because they are more nutritious. They can be consumed occasionally if handled in the right way, that is, soaked and washed prior to cooking them. The "pseudograins" to avoid on a Paleo diet:

- quinoa
- amaranth
- chia seeds
- buckwheat

- hemp (seeds and plant)
- flax (seeds and plant)

Dairy doesn't seem to be much of an issue with a Paleo diet, although there are many studies out there that will tell you how cow's milk is linked to gut inflammation, allergies and asthma – to name only a few. It's particularly the protein in cow's milk called 'casein' that people who are lactose intolerant cannot digest. In the Paleo diet, dairy is said to be consumed in moderate amounts, including: ghee, butter, kefir (fermented milk), cream, ricotta, halloumi, feta, aged cheeses like pecorino, cheddar and parmesan, and goat's cheeses.

Nuts and seeds in the Paleo perspective are said to be high in pro-inflammatory omega-6 fatty acids as well as anti-nutrients such as phytic acid and enzyme inhibitors, which prevent the absorption of minerals in the body. Paleo enthusiasts recommend soaking nuts and seeds for 6-12 hours in water, then dehydrate them in sunlight, a dehydrator machine, or in the oven. That way, the high percentage of anti-nutrients are largely removed.

Vegetarian

Vegetarians don't consume meat or anything that has 'died' in the strictest sense. Cow milk, sheep's milk, dairy products such as butter and yogurt, and honey are consumed by vegetarians. Some vegetarians don't consume cow milk because often the mother cow's child (the calf) is taken away shortly after birth and given either a milk replacement, or is killed. The milk the cow produces naturally for her child is then harvested commercially and sold in stores for human consumption. This is the case for dairy cows, not cattle being raised to eat. Dairy cows are injected with so many growth hormones that I personally doubt their flesh would be allowed for human consumption.

Interesting fact: Humans are the only animals known to drink milk from another species, and also well after the early periods of growth in their lives.

Vegetarians also don't eat gelatine because that food product comes from bones / bone marrow of animals, and to harvest that, the animals must be slaughtered.

Lacto-Ovotarian

This group is similar to vegetarians, except they do eat eggs and milk. Hence 'lacto', which is short for 'lactose', the protein found in animal milk. And 'ovo' is Latin for 'egg'.

Pescatarian

These are vegetarians who eat fish, but don't eat other meats such as poultry, chicken, beef, pork or other animal meats. The premise is that fish are one of the best sources of omega 3, 6, and 9 fatty acids.

Fruitarian

Fruitarians believe in only eating the fruit of a plant, tree, or shrub. The premise is to cause no harm to plants as well as animals, so they wouldn't harvest grain or corn, for example; they would only eat fruit that falls from the tree or vine. This also includes seeds and nuts.

This diet, as you can imagine, includes considerable danger to one's health if the body isn't prepared for this kind of diet, and if the Fruitarian doesn't take extra caution to consume the recommended amounts of vitamins and minerals.

Some fruitarians choose their diet out of a moral and ethical ground. Others, similar to Paleo dieters, believe that humans were hunter-gatherers before agrarian society distorted social structure and humans' way of life, and so they choose to live in the 'natural state' of early man, but with a modern, evolved twist that no animal must be or should be killed.

Veganism

Vegans are very similar to vegetarians, except that they choose to not consume *any* animal-based products. This excludes cow milk, sheep's milk, goat's milk (and the like), butters made from the former, eggs, gelatine and honey. Usually, vegans also exclude products from their lives that have caused harm to animals, for example, leather shoes or cosmetics that have been tested on animals.

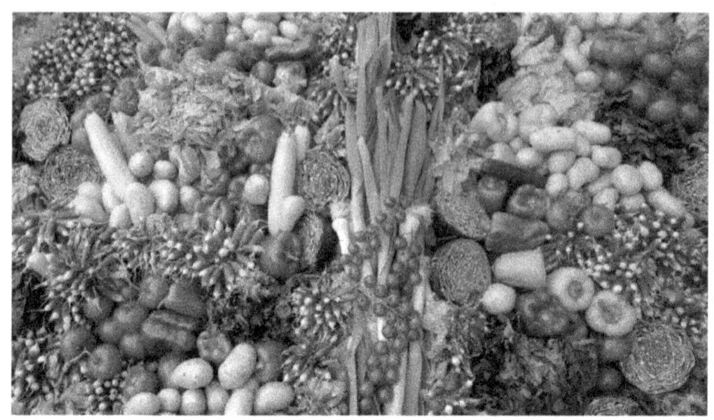

[2] Staples of a Plant-Based Diet

I'm often skeptical of new foods and fads that seems to sweep the nation (or at least the Internet and my Instagram feed). When I analyze their nutritional content, they seem very ordinary -- take goji berries, for example. They're difficult to find fresh, and the dried berries taste very similar to blueberries in that they're less tart in flavor. Figs and apricots also have a smooth taste, and are half the price of these 'super foods' imported from South America.

Before going crazy for a new superfood or fad, consider the impact is has on your gut -- does it have higher vitamin or mineral content? Does it have a good amount of omega fatty acids? -- and then consider the impact it has on the environment: does the produce or food have to be shipped from far away, like Perú or Thailand, in order to end up in your kitchen? What's the carbon emissions impact of such a long journey for a bit of food? Not only is food less ripe when travelling such a long distance, but it usually has less nutritional content because it's not ripe when picked or harvested.

[2.1] Fruits & Vegetables

The Encyclopedia of Healing Foods (see Appendix D) states that "regular fruit consumption may also help control the appetite and promote weight loss. While aspartame (NutraSweet), glucose, and sucrose may increase the appetite, fructose has actually been shown to decrease the amount of calories and fat consumed in several studies." It hails fruit as an excellent snack in between meals because many studies mentioned involved consuming this natural fruit sugar 30 to 60 minutes prior to eating a meal.

Here are a few staples that are easy to find anywhere across the States in grocery stores:

- **Apples** - It's a member of the rose family, just like pears. There are over 7,000 varieties. In Norse mythology, they were believed to keep people young forever. Most of the apple's important nutrients are contained in its skin. One small serving of an apple (appx 3.5 ounces) is a small apple fitting comfortably in your hand, and has 52 calories, 2.4 grams of fiber, and 10.4 grams of natural sugars. Its real value lies in many minerals and phytochemicals such as ellagic acid and flavonoids like quercetin -- those don't sound appealing, and the complex names don't often make it into magazine headlines for this reason.

- **Avocados** - They're an excellent source of monounsaturated fatty acids, potassium, Vitamin E, B vitamins, and fiber. Fun fact: one avocado has the same potassium content of 2-3 bananas!

- **Beets** or 'beetroots' are rich in calcium, iron, vitamins A and C. Their green, leafy stalks can be eaten in salads and soups. They've long been used medicinally to stimulate a healthy liver and promote natural detoxification.

- **Carrots** - The leafy green tops of carrots can also be eaten, though their bitter taste is more suitable for a soup or stew than a salad. Carrots are very high in Vitamin A, which is good for your eyes. Two carrots provide four times the recommended daily allowance of vitamin A. They also have vitamin K, biotin, and fiber. Fun fact: carrots were originally purple on the outside and orange on the inside.

- **Dates** - Some cultures call date trees the "Tree of Life", most likely for their ability to withstand drought and that their fruits gave instant sugary sustenance. Dates are a very alkaline food and are high in fiber -- the better kind of fiber, in fact, that passes through the intestinal tract more slowly than insoluble fiber. Dates can actually - contrary to most uneducated beliefs - aid in weight loss because their fiber content slows down gastric emptying (when your stomach passes on its contents to the next in line to process food), thereby leaving to a feeling of satiation and a satisfied 'fullness'.

- **Lemons** are extremely high in Vitamin C, which has been known to prevent tumor growth and cure a number of other illnesses. Lemons are the only fruit that doesn't curdle in boiling water, which is why lemon is often added to tea. Some cultures, like in Russia or Tajikistan, add marmelade to their tea instead of fresh lemon (which can be expensive).

[2.2] Seeds & Nuts

- **Almonds** - high in fat, just 3.5 ounces (enough to make a scant handful) has 600 calories. They are packed with nutrition, however, with 20% protein, potassium, magnesium, calcium, iron, zinc, and vitamin E. They also have antioxidant flavonoids, to stave off cancer and other illnesses.

- **Chia seeds** - these contain all the amino acids we need to build protein. They're best consumed after sitting in water for 10-20 minutes, when they start to sprout and little translucent bubbles appear around the edges, looking very similar to human blood cells.

- **Flaxseeds** - also called Linseeds, these were so beloved by Charlemagne in the 8th century C.E. (or after Christ's Death, a.k.a. A.D.) that he passed laws and regulations requiring his subjects consume flaxseeds. They are high in omega 3 fatty acids, phosphorous, iron, and copper. They contain nearly twice the level of omega 3 as fish oil, but it's short-chain acids rather than the long-chain in fish oil.

- **Olives** - olives are technically a fruit, and their high fat content (15-35%) is shown to be the 'good' kind which prevents heart disease and chronic conditions.

[2.3] Grains & Legumes

- **Barley** - is likely the oldest grain known to our record-keeping civilizations, being cultivated as long ago as 8,000 B.C.E. It has virtually the same nutritional elements as corn, being a good source of fiber and selenium, copper, magnesium and phosphorous.

- **Soybeans** - many sources use scare tactics with little facts behind them to make people think that the synthetic form of plant estrogen in soy can throw off a woman's reproductive cycle or hormonal balance. This is, in truth, hardly ever the case if at all -- only women who have estrogen-sensitive breast tumors (not anywhere else) should restrict their soy intake to 4 servings per week. No conclusive studies have been done proving this. The only real 'bad' characteristic about soy is that the farmers who harvest it in South America are often not paid fairly, and the beans consume copious amounts of water, and oil-based products in order to be transported into the U.S. <u>The Encyclopedia of Natural Medicine</u> states "the benefits of soy could fill a large book. It is one of the world's most important foods," citing its high protein content, essential fatty acids and fiber.

- **Lentils** - they have roughly the same nutritional content as common beans, being a good source of protein, dietary fiber (which lowers cholesterol) and folic acid.

[2.4] "Interesting" Foods

- **Honey** - is a good source of riboflavin, iron, manganese, and vitamin B6. It's very high in sugar content, with bee pollen actually containing complete proteins with all amino acids needed to build protein in humans.

- **Mushrooms** - depending on the variety, are an excellent source of many minerals like copper, selenium, potassium and zinc. They're also very high in many B Vitamins. They have zero cholesterol, are high in fiber and very low in calories, with about 22 calories in a 3.5-ounce serving.

- **Seaweed** or "sea vegetables" - contain literally all the minerals found in the ocean, which are the exact same minerals found in human blood. A variety of seaweed provides an excellent source of *all* these minerals like calcium iodine, sodium, magnesium, iron, potassium, and riboflavin, just to name a few.

[2.5] Nutritional Supplements to Support Your Plant-Based Diet

As mentioned earlier in Chapter One, it's important to be aware of your iron and B12 consumption. **Iron** can often be consumed from plant sources, but women of child-bearing age might want to take iron supplements during their menstruation, as iron is lost in blood and blood clots. Be careful not to consume too much iron, as that can cause bloating and constipation.

B12 supplements are easy to find online or in your local drug store. Often, you'll find the B Vitamin family together in one supplement along with Vitamin C and a few others. It's fine to take these 'broad-ranging' supplements. Be sure to switch manufacturers often, so that your body does not grow accustomed to one type of synthetic supplement and then slowly start to absorb less and less.

Protein is often an issue with vegans who are between pubescent age and their mid-forties. I've found a vegan pea protein isolate that tastes, well, a bit like cardboard but can easily slip into a soup, stew, sauce, or smoothie unnoticed. Be careful to read the labels of protein bars -- some are actually quite low in protein, and others contain milk, or whey protein (from milk), or harmful additives and colorants / dyes. The best way to boost your protein is by drinking a smoothie with banana, chia seeds, soy milk, and pea protein powder. I usually sweeten mine up with peanut butter or honey / agave syrup too.

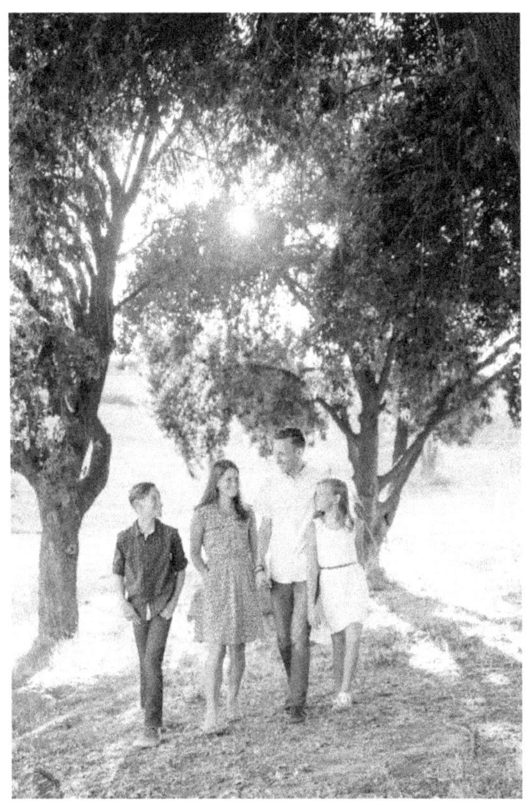

[3] Health Benefits & Disease Prevention Or Reversal

This was briefly mentioned in the overview in Chapter One. The book <u>Encyclopedia of Natural Medicine</u> referenced in Appendix D is simply a life-saver if you'd like to read up more on these individual topics.

Re-Balancing the Body's pH

Refined sugar and simple carbohydrates (like in donuts, white bread, and the rest) tend to make the body more acidic. All sorts of chronic illnesses and diseases flourish in an acidic state, including candida overgrown, arthritis, cancers, and tumors. Here's a list of alkaline foods:

- Arugula
- Asparagus
- Avocados
- Bananas and other fruit of your choice for smoothies
- Beets / beetroot
- Broccoli
- Cabbage
- Carrots
- Cauliflower
- Celery
- Cucumber
- Eggplant
- Fennel
- Fresh herbs
- Garlic
- Ginger root
- Grapefruit
- Green apples
- Green beans
- Jalapeño peppers
- Kale
- Lemons
- Limes
- Onions
- Other leafy greens (collards, bok choy, escarole, etc.)
- Parsnips
- Radishes
- Red, yellow bell peppers
- Romaine
- Shallots
- Snap peas, snow peas
- Spaghetti squash
- Spinach
- Sprouts
- Sweet potatoes

- Swiss chard
- Tomatoes
- Watercress
- Yellow squash
- Zucchini

A Few Specific Diseases

Gout specifically can be cured and prevented with a plant-based diet. Gout is the result of increased synthesis of uric acid, or the reduced ability to excrete uric acid. Alternatively, there can be overproduction of uric acid and your body isn't able to excrete it in the urine fast enough. To cure gout, avoid and eliminate:

- Alcohol
- Organ meats, meat, poultry
- Yeast
- Refined carbs
- Excessive calories

A low fat and protein intake also helps considerably. Increase your consumption of alkaline foods like celery, cherries, and blueberries.

Asthma can be triggered and made worse by Yellow Dye #5 which is often found in processed foods but already banned in many European countries. Milk products (cow milk, that is) have been linked to an increase of phlegm and acidity in the body, which worsens asthma, allergies, and hay fever.

Hypertension or 'high blood pressure' as it's more commonly known, is a serious problem in the UK and the US. A normal blood pressure is around 120 over 80. Anything above this level signifies a major risk factor for heart attack and stroke. Caffeine, alcohol, and tobacco should be eliminated. Natural stress reduction techniques such as biofeedback, bioresonance, yoga, meditation and autogenics can help lower blood pressure. Celery seed extract has been known to lower high blood pressure and anti-ACE peptides as well. Eat a diet low in sodium -- 200 mg a day is the minimum recommended allowance -- and high in potassium. Increase your intake of fruits, veggies, whole grains and legumes.

No Sugar, Less Crime?

We all know that refined sugar is bad for us, but could it actually make our behavior bad as well as our teeth? The book "Food for Thought" (Miller & Miller) points out a very shocking correlation between consumption of white sugar and criminal behavior. "Low blood sugar," they posit in <u>Food for Thought,</u> "which is becoming widespread, has been directly correlated with all sorts of criminal behavior. The list includes assault, arson, murder, robbery and vandalism. In one Argentinian study, blood-sugar tests were taken on a group of one hundred and twenty-nine apprehended delinquents. Only thirteen were reported to have had blood sugars within the normal limits."

There are numerous other studies that have been conducted largely in the USA, noting the effects of hypoglycemia (low blood sugar) on violent and criminal behavior, including marital conflicts and domestic violence. As early as 1974 Dick Gregory, a somewhat well-known American personality at the time, published a diet book stating:

"As a veteran occupant of some of the nation's most prestigious jails, I think the jails and prisons of America would be a perfect place to initiate dietary reform and nutritional rehabilitation. In the jails are many addicts and others suffering from mental disturbance and emotional hostilities which could be corrected by dietary reform."

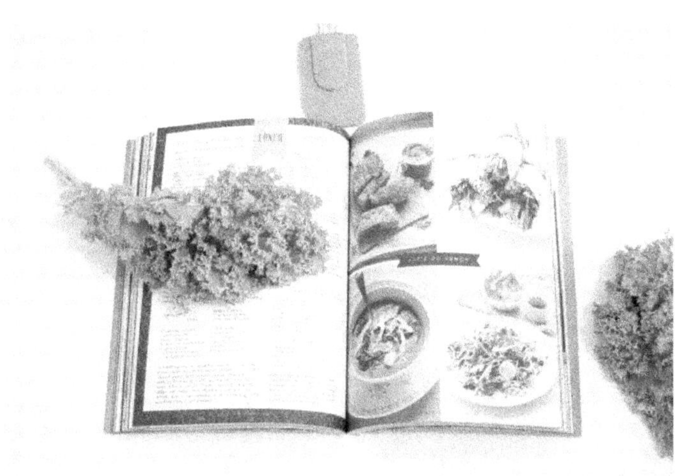

[4] Recipes

All recipes focus on packing your mealtime or snack with macronutrients and tasty, creative alternatives to store-bought, packaged food.

I've arranged the recipes here by meal / mealtime / snack, which fit nicely into the meal plans coming up in the next chapter.

[4.1] Breakfast

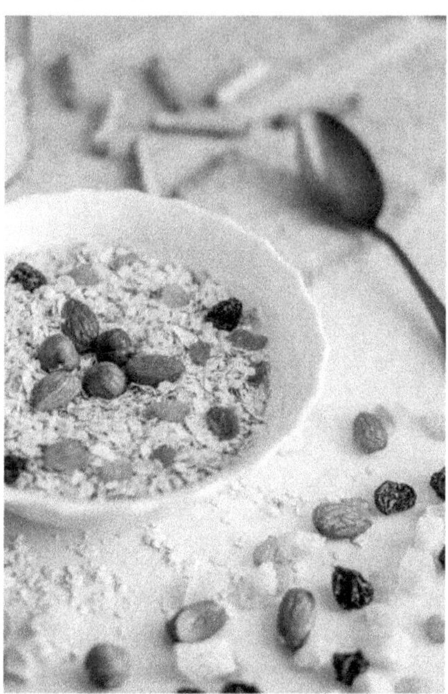

High Protein Oatmeal with Chia Seeds & Almonds

Prep time: 5 min.

Cook time: 10 min.

Storage time: Up to 8 days in the fridge or 3 months in the freezer

Suitable diets: Gluten-Free, Vegan, Vegetarian

Calories: 298 kcal

Protein: 10.3 g

Carbs: 35.3 g

Fat: 14.4 g

Makes: three adult-sized servings

Ingredients:
- 3 cups Unsweetened Almond Milk
- 1 ½ cup Old Fashioned Oats (Quaker Oats for example – just anything that isn't instant)

- 3 tablespoons chia seeds, more to sprinkle on top if you'd like
- 4–6 tablespoons unsalted nuts (hazelnuts, walnuts, almonds, macadamia nuts, etc.)
- 6 tablespoons dried or fresh fruit (For the one you see in the picture I used mulberries and pomegranate)

Instructions:

Place almond milk, oats, chia seeds, and nuts in a small saucepan and let it come to a boil. Reduce heat after bringing to a boil. Cook for about 5-9 minutes over medium heat, stirring occasionally. Place it in a bowl and garnish it with more nuts, dried fruits and chia seeds, if preferred.

Variations:

- Vegetarian – use cow milk if you'd like, substituted one to one
- Raw – this is perfect for raw food enthusiasts; simply mix all ingredients together, adding 1 more cup of water, because the chia seeds soak up a lot of liquid. Let sit in the fridge overnight, and enjoy in the morning!

Savory Golden Oatmeal

Yes, oats can be savory! They make a delicious, almost creamy base for any breakfast food. So if you're like me and prefer something more hearty than sugary and sweet first thing in the morning, this is the perfect recipe for you.

Prep time: 5 min.
Cook time: 10 min.
Storage time: Up to 7 days in the fridge
Suitable diets: Gluten-Free, Vegan, Vegetarian

Calories: 238 kcal
Protein: 9 g
Carbs: 34 g
Fat: 7,2 g (of which 2.4 g saturates)
Makes: 2 adult-sized servings

Ingredients:
- 1 clove garlic, minced
- ½ cup carrots, grated
- 2 tablespoon(s) roasted red bell peppers
- ¼ teaspoon(s) turmeric
- ½ tablespoon(s) fresh herbs such as dill or basil, plus more if you'd like for garnish
- 1 tablespoon(s) vegan cream cheese
- 2 ½ cup low-sodium vegetable broth
- 1 cup rolled oats or quick / instant oats
- Salt and pepper to taste

Instructions:
Pour just a splash of the veggie broth (not all of it) into a medium sized pot. Add the minced garlic and sauté over medium heat for 2-3 minutes, or until translucent.

Pour in more vegetable broth (also called 'soup stock' sometimes) and then add the carrots, red pepper, herbs and tumeric. Let cook for 2-3 minutes before stirring in the vegan cream cheese. Stir until it's even and smooth, and be careful it doesn't burn.

Next, add the oats and the rest of the vegetable broth to the pot. Increase the heat to high until the mixture starts to boil, then turn the heat back down to medium and cook until your desired consistency is reached, stirring frequently.

Transfer the savory oatmeal into two bowls and sprinkle more fresh herbs on top, and maybe a drizzle of your favorite nut butter.

Not-So-Traditional Polish Potato Pancakes

These take a much healthier, modern spin on the traditional potato pancakes (called *Latkes*) that originated in Poland. Rather than using eggs, I've devised a combination of vegan ingredients that work quite well to hold the mixture together. And they're naturally gluten-free – although some versions I've seen do add a bit of flour for whatever reason.

Prep time: 20 min.
Cook time: 15 min.
Storage time: Up to 7 days in the fridge
Suitable diets: Gluten-Free, Vegan, Vegetarian

Calories: 41 kcal (that's not a typo!)
Protein: 1 g
Carbs: 5 g
Fat: 1.2 g (of which 0.3 g saturates)
Makes: 15 pancakes

Ingredients:
- 1 pound potatoes
- 3 Tablespoons tapioca flour
- 3 Tablespoons blanched almond flour
- 2 Tablespoons ground flax seeds (also called "flax meal")
- 3/4 teaspoon onion powder
- 2 teaspoons avocado oil or walnut oil + more for frying

Instructions:
Wash and grate your potatoes. You can peel them if you prefer a smoother texture to your potato pancakes, but most of the nutrients are in the peel so I'd advise leaving it on.

While you heat up a large skillet or frying pan, let the grated pile of potatoes sit for a couple minutes, so that the water mostly starts to pool at the bottom. Then, wrap them in a clean kitchen towel and press out as much water as you can. Don't go overboard, because these don't need to be ultra-dry. Less moisture simply helps the pancakes stick together.

In a medium-sized bowl, mix together the almond flour, tapioca flour, onion powder and ground flax seeds. Add the potatoes, and toss to ensure they're well coated in the mixture.

Add the oil and mix well. (Note: You can use olive oil or veggie oil, but I like the taste of the two I've suggested above.)

By now, your frying pan should be well heated up. Pour enough oil into the pan to cover the bottom by about one half inch. You want to slightly (deep fat) fry them, but not inundated them completely into the oil like you would a donut. Tidy up the kitchen a bit as you wait for the oil to heat.

Use a large serving spoon or an ice cream scoop to portion out the pancakes. Roll the portions into a ball first, then press into a pancake, and gently place the pancakes into the frying pan.

Cook for 3-5 minutes, or until the bottom has taken on a deep golden brown color. Flip them over and cook until the other side reaches the same color.

Take a large plate or serving tray and line with a few clean paper towels or kitchen towels (if you enjoy washing oil out of linens!) Remove the pancakes from the pan and place them onto the plate. Let the excess oil drain out. Eat immediately while they are still warm. Some of my family's favorites include applesauce, vegan sour cream, chopped fresh herbs, and nut butter.

Oven-Roasted Breakfast Potatoes

"Baking potatoes" (the large white ones that are usually labeled as 'for baking') usually don't have much flavor on their own; that's why I use them in soups or mixed into a casserole as a "base" or place-holder for some substance. There are lots of cute, tasty little potatoes that you can find if you look around at co-ops and other more alternative stores. Or, some large grocery stores may have a wider variety as well. The quality definitely makes a difference in this recipe!

This is also a perfect party recipe, because people can eat it easily with a toothpick or dip it into homemade hummus or olive spread. They're best served hot, but don't lose their delicious flavor when cooled, such as at a party.

Prep time: 40 min.
Cook time: 45 min.
Storage time: Up to 8 days in the fridge
Suitable diets: Gluten-Free, Vegan, Vegetarian, Paleo

Calories: 160 kcal
Protein: 4 g
Carbs: 21 g
Fat: 11.2 g (1.3 grams of which saturates)
Makes: 4 servings (of a small-ish portion, they're either for breakfast or meant as a side dish)

Ingredients:

- 1.5 pounds of yellow potatoes
- 3 Tablespoons olive oil
- ½ teaspoon Himalaya salt
- 1 teaspoon dried rosemary or 2 teaspoons freshly chopped rosemary
- ½ teaspoon dried thyme or 1 teaspoon freshly chopped thyme

Instructions:

Cut the potatoes into large, bite-sized pieces. Soak the potatoes in a large bowl of ice water for 20-30 minutes.

While the potatoes soak, chop your fresh herbs. If you're using dried, this is a great time to soak the dried herbs in the olive oil (in a shot glass or other small, small bowl) in order to bring out their flavor and soften the dried herbs. Especially rosemary can be similar to pine needs, long and pointy and kind of sharp to bite into from the wrong angle!

Add the herbs, olive oil, and salt into a small bowl and mix well. Add pepper to taste. (I don't recommend it, because it distracts from the delicious, dark taste of the herbs.)

Preheat your oven to 450°F or gas mark 6.

Drain the water from the potatoes and spread them out onto a kitchen towel. Use another towel to pat them dry. This removes much of the starch from potatoes, which makes them chewier, almost tougher – think of potato starch as an ingredient in soup stocks to thicken it. *That's* why you soak and drain them!

Transfer the potatoes into two large cast iron pans or baking sheets lined with tin foil or wax paper. Bake for 30 minutes. Flip them, then bake for another 15 minutes or until crispy on all sides.

<u>Storage Tip</u>: Reheat in the oven to keep their crispy texture. Microwaves tend to distort the texture of some root vegetables.

Potatoes, like varieties of white rice, don't seem to freeze well. After they're thawed, they take on a different texture. If you'd like to use up these potatoes when they've been hanging out in the back of your fridge for a week – lest they be thrown in the trash! - it's easy enough to add 1 cup of water, 1 tablespoon of soup stock, blend well, and throw in the freezer. Voila! You can use this to 'pad out' or 'thicken up' a soup you'll cook in the future.

Cinnamon Almond Breakfast Muffins

Don't be daunted by the long ingredient list! I made this recipe by pure experiment, adding a bit of things here and there until I achieved the right consistency of a vegan muffin.

This is a delicious recipe I made up when experimenting one day. I don't seem to find many recipes combining apple and almond for some reason. If you don't like the combination of the two mild flavors together, then feel free to substitute the apple for half of a large zucchini, which would add the same amount of moisture to the recipe but without the recognizable flavor of apple.

I recommend eating these warm with almond nut butter and some chopped almonds sprinkled on top. They do freeze quite well, also.

Prep time: 25 min.
Bake time: 25 min.
Storage time: Up to 6 days in an airtight container or 6 months in the freezer
Suitable diets: Gluten-Free, Vegan, Vegetarian

Calories: 224 kcal
Protein: 4 g
Carbs: 30 g
Fat: 9 g (1 gram of which saturates)
Makes: 12 muffins

Ingredients:
- ¾ cup muesli / oat granola mix
- 1 cup plain flour (unpacked)
- 1 teaspoon baking powder
- 1 teaspoon baking soda
- 1 teaspoon cinnamon
- 2 pinches of nutmeg
- 1 pinch of Himalaya salt
- ¼ cup light brown soft sugar
- ½ teaspoon almond extract
- 1 teaspoon white wine vinegar or apple cider vinegar

- 1 ¼ cup sweetened almond milk (or soy / hazelnut / oat milk)
  Or, if you like the apple flavor, use ¾ cup almond milk and ½ cup apple juice
- 1 fresh red apple (or ½ large zucchini)
- 2 tablespoon(s) grapeseed oil (or avocado, peanut, sesame or walnut oil)
- 3 tablespoon(s) almond nut butter
- 4 tablespoon(s) sugar or granulated stevia
- ½ cup ground almonds
- ½ cup chopped almonds (and flaked or sliced almonds on top, if you wish)

Instructions:

Heat the oven to 400°F or 370°F fan or gas mark 6. Line a muffin tin with cases. I recommend using silicon cases which are reusable and let the muffins slide / pop out when cooled very easily. Alternatively, you can grease the muffin tin with veggie margarine and sprinkle a little flour on top to ensure the muffins slide out of the tin well enough.

Mix the dry ingredients together, ensuring they are blended well. Then, pour in the muesli / granola and mix. Add the rest of the wet ingredients (including sugar, because it technically is considered a moist ingredient), making sure to stir the almond extract into the mixture well, otherwise you'll get a surprise bit of too much almond!

Note: It's absolutely okay to see small bubbles (smaller than an apple seed) bubbling up from the mixture. That's the chemical reaction between the vinegar and baking soda, which makes the muffins more light and fluffy in texture.

Divide the mixture equally between the 12 muffin cases. They should be between about three-quarters and 90% full. Any more mixture, and it will bubble over and burn while baking.

Bake in the middle rack of the oven for 25-30 minutes or until they've risen and are golden brown. Cool in tins / cases / silicone muffin cases outside the oven.

Apple Cinnamon French Toast

Yes, a delicious French Toast can be made without eggs and cow's milk! It's a sweet favorite with apples, berries or bananas – or you can enjoy it with nut butter and a sprinkling of chopped nuts atop.

Food Saver Tip: If you have bread that is drying out or nearing its expiry date, throw it in the freezer to keep it for another 3-4 months. It can be thawed quickly and easily in the toaster. And if it's too old and dried out? Transform it into a delicious French Toast!

Prep time: 20 min.
Bake time: 20 min.
Storage time: Up to 3 days in an airtight container
Suitable diets: Vegan, Vegetarian

Calories: 210 kcal*
Protein: 5 g
Carbs: 32 g
Fat: 6 g (1 gram of which saturates)
Makes: 6 servings / slices
The exact amount of calories depends on the type of bread you choose to use.

Ingredients:

- 3 tablespoons maple syrup
- 1 medium-sized apple
- 2 tablespoon(s) flour
- 2 tablespoon(s) ground almonds
- 2 teaspoon(s) cinnamon
- 200ml oat milk or rice milk
- 1 tablespoon(s) white sugar
- 1 teaspoon(s) vanilla extract
- 6 slices of thick white bread
- Oil for frying (choose a light one like vegetable, sunflower, walnut or grapeseed)
- Powdered sugar (also called "icing sugar" for dusting on top)

Instructions:

Wash and cut the apple into quarters. Some prefer to peel the apple, but I leave the peel on if it's unwaxed and organic, because the peel includes many health-restoring nutrients. The adage "an apple a day keeps the doctor away" was coined in a time when people didn't have the luxury of being able to peel apples and waste any food!

Finely grate or shred one quarter of the apple, adding it and the maple syrup and the cinnamon into a saucepan. Bring gently to a medium heat, stirring often to avoid burning and mixing the cinnamon well. (The heat brings out more of its flavor.)

Whisk together the flour, ground almonds, milk and vanilla extract together in a shallow bowl. Add the cooked apple mixture and blend well. If you don't have a shallow bowl, then pour the mixture into a deep plate or cake pan.

Place 6 slices of bread in the mixture and give them a minute to soak up the delicious batter while you heat a small amount of oil in a frying pan on medium heat or gas mark 4. Flip the slices of bread so that the other side can soak up the French Toast batter.

Shake off excess batter before placing them in the pan to fry. 2-4 minutes should give you a nice medium, golden brown on one edge. Flip the slices and cook another 2-3 minutes. It should look crispy and brown on the edges and in the middle.

Keep the slices warm in the oven at low heat as you fry the rest of the slices. Chop the remaining three quarters of the apple, sprinkling it and powdered sugar on top of the French Toast to serve.

[4.2] Salads

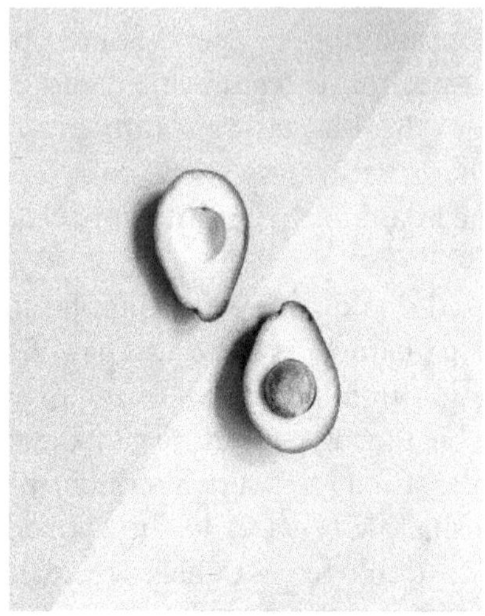

Avocado & Tofu Scramble

This is a super-easy recipe to throw together, and always reminds me of a lazy Sunday morning when the kids are playing quietly, my beautiful partner brings me coffee in bed, and nothing's planned for the day. This scramble can easily be made for brunch because the avocado makes it a bit more filling.

<u>Food Saver Tip</u>: If you'd like your avocado to not go brown after a few hours, sprinkle lemon juice on top. The high vitamin C content in lemon juice keeps the vitamin C from breaking down right away and causing your avocado to turn brown. This trick also works well with apples.

Prep time: 10 min.
Cook time: 6-7 min.
Storage time: Up to 1 day in an airtight container (storing in the fridge would make the water separate from the mixture more, distorting its consistency)
Suitable diets: Vegan, Vegetarian, Paleo, Low-Sugar

Calories: 358 kcal*
Protein: 17.5 g

Carbs: 7.3 g
Fat: 27.5 g (1.1 gram of which saturates)
Makes: 4 servings

Ingredients:

- 2 tablespoons extra virgin olive oil
- 1 onion (yellow or white)
- 4 garlic cloves
- 1-2 red chillies (depending on how spicy you like it)
- 1 zucchini
- 1 teaspoon smoked paprika
- 1 teaspoon ground cumin
- 1 teaspoon dried oregano
- 2-3 handfuls of spinach
- 1 package (450g or 16 ounces) smoked tofu
- 4 pieces of toasted bread to serve (sourdough or the gluten-free, Paleo-friendly recipe included later in this book)
- 1 large avocado (stays fresh and tasty if you sprinkle lime juice over it)
- ½ bunch of cilantro / coriander to serve

Instructions:

Heat the olive oil in a frying pan on medium heat as you chop the garlic, chop the zucchini, finely chop the chili and press the onion. Add those to the frying pan all at once and cook for about 4 minutes or until they've started to soften.

Meanwhile, put the tofu into a bowl and mash it until it looks like scrambled eggs. Stir this into the pan before you throw in the seasonings listed above, stirring well, and cook for another 2 minutes.

After everything is fully heated, add the spinach and toss for another few minutes until wilted. If you have an electric stovetop, turn off the heat just before you add in the spinach and it'll reach the perfect 'just-cooked-enough' texture. (Remember, the more you cook vegetables, the more vitamins you lose!) Serve with toast, tortilla, or bread of your choice with avocado and chopped cilantro.

Roasted Sweet Potato & Almond Salad

Freekeh, also called Farik, is similar to couscous in that it's a small, round grain used as a staple in Middle Eastern (specifically Levantine and Northern African) dishes. It is roasted and rubbed apart, giving it a distinct flavor somewhat reminiscent of barley (with that 'roasted' flavor).

If you don't want to make it yourself or cannot find it, simply replace it one-to-one with couscous, bulgur, or millet.

Prep time: 15 min.
Bake time: 35 min.
Storage time: Up to 1 day in an airtight container in the fridge (keep the rocket separate to prevent wilting)
Suitable diets: Gluten-Free, Vegan, Vegetarian, Paleo

Calories: 430 kcal
Protein: 12 g
Carbs: 66.8 g
Fat: 9.7 g (1.3 grams of which saturates)
Makes: 3 portions

Ingredients:
- 2 medium sweet potatoes
- 2 teaspoons coriander seeds
- 2 teaspoons cumin seeds
- 1 tablespoon vegetable or walnut oil
- 1 ½ cup pre-cooked freekeh
- 1 handful of rocket
- ½ bunch of coriander (approximately one heaping half cup when chopped)

HARISSA YOGURT DRESSING
- 3 tablespoons of low-fat greek style soy yogurt
- 1 tablespoon rose harissa
- 1 fresh lemon (or 5 tablespoons of lemon juice)

Instructions:

Heat the oven to 400°F / 370°F fan / gas mark 6. Wash and chop the sweet potato, leaving the skins on if you prefer. Toss the sweet potato with the spices and oil, and place them flat on a baking tray.

Bake the potato blend for 30-35 minutes or until the sweet potato is very soft when poked with a fork and charred at the edges.

Heat the freekeh following pack instructions and tip into a bowl with the sweet potato. Whisk the dressing ingredients with 1-2 tablespoons of cold water, until it's got a consistency that is liquid enough to drizzle on the salad but also thick enough to not be runny and 'escape' from flavoring the salad.

Add the rocket, coriander and ⅔ of the dressing to the freekeh and sweet potato, and gently mix. Serve and drizzle with the remaining dressing on top.

Crunchy, Protein-Packed Salad with Chili Dressing

Prep time: 15 min.
Cook time: 0 min.
Storage time: Up to 1 day in an airtight container in the fridge (keep the rocket separate to prevent wilting)
Suitable diets: Gluten-Free, Vegan, Vegetarian, Paleo, Low-Sugar

Calories: 201 kcal
Protein: 10.2 g
Carbs: 20.8 g
Fat: 9.8 g (1.6 grams of which saturates)
Makes: 2 portions

Ingredients:

- 4 celery stalks
- 2 cups green beans
- ½ 8-ounce block firm tofu
- ¼ cup unsalted, roasted peanuts
- 2 tablespoons lime juice
- 2 tablespoons Chile Crisp
- Himalaya or sea salt and pepper to taste

Instructions:

Trim the celery stalks and cut off the white, round parts on the bottom (they don't taste very good). Save them for putting in a soup, or composting. Trim the tips off the green beans and slice at a steep diagonal into bite-sized pieces. Slice the tofu into thin batons or strips.

Toss the celery, green beans, tofu, peanuts, lime juice, and chili crisp (or chili flakes) in a medium bowl to combine well. Add salt and pepper to taste, serving chilled.

Marinated Tofu with Pickled Spring Vegetables

Marination is an easy way to add some flavor to any staple food: potatoes, tofu, onions, or meat (if you're cooking for meat eaters). So is pickling. It's surprisingly easy to do at home (read the section on Storage in this book) and produce tends to be more crisp and flavorful when pickled at home.

Prep time: overnight (for the marination) + 15 minutes
Cook time: 5 min
Storage time: 2 days in the fridge (if you keep the fresh cilantro separate)
Suitable diets: Vegan, Vegetarian, Gluten-Free, Paleo

Calories: 142 kcal
Protein: 12.4 g
Carbs: 11.7 g
Fat: 6.3 g (1.2 grams of which saturates)
Makes: 4 portions

Ingredients:

- 12 sugar snap peas
- 12 snow peas (also called "mangetouts")
- 1 bunch of asparagus
- 2 tablespoons white sugar-fr1/3 cup rice vinegar (although any kind will do)
- 1 small white radish (also called "daikon")
- 6-8 scallions / spring onions
- 1 small bunch of cilantro / coriander
- 6 tablespoons Bragg's Amino Acids or light soy sauce
- 2 dashes of sesame oil
- 1 tablespoon sesame seeds
- ½ teaspoon Chinese five-spice powder
- 1 pound firm tofu (sold in one big block)

Instructions:

To make the marinated tofu, you'll need to put 3 tablespoons of Bragg's Amino Acids together with the Chinese five-spice powder and the tofu in a bowl. If it doesn't fit snugly enough, what I do is add a dash of water to thin out the marinade and spread it out in a small baking dish. I slice the tofu into thin slices and lay in the marinade. Cover well so no air gets in, and let sit overnight (usually in the fridge, but on the counter top is also okay.) Turn the tofu over every few hours if you can.

The next day, remove the tofu from the marinade and set aside. Cut the asparagus into bite-sized lengths of 1-2 inches, and trip the bitter, white-ish bottoms from the asparagus.

Take a saucepan with lightly salted water and bring it to a boil. Add the asparagus, sugar snap peas and snow peas, which you might want to cut in half lengthwise. Blanch them (cook them on high heat) for 1 minute. Drain and place into a large bowl of ice water until they are completely cold. Drain well and place into another medium-sized bowl.

Put the sugar and vinegar into a small saucepan and boil for 5 minutes, until it's thickened just a little. Remove from the heat and let the mixture cool down. Pour the mixture over the blanched vegetables and daikon, stir well, and set aside for half an hour.

Add the sliced spring onions, cilantro / coriander, and marinated tofu to the pickled vegetables, gently tossing to combine.

Mix in the rest of the Bragg's Amino Acids (3 tablespoons) and the sesame oil together in a small bowl. Pour over the salad. Toss gently, then transfer to a serving dish and sprinkle the sesame seeds over the top, toasting them beforehand if you'd like. (This is done on medium low heat in a frying pan, without oil, for about 10 minutes or until they've turned a nice medium golden brown color.)

53

Cashew Salad with Tamarind Dressing

This is a delightful, tasty salad with south-east Asian flavor. Tamarind looks something similar to peanuts with its hard outer shell that's thinner and more of a dark brown color. It has large seeds inside, and a very sugary sweet, slightly sour flesh. In its fresh form, it's simply delicious. Tamarind is commonly found in Asia and the Middle East. If you cannot find any Tamarind in your local supermarket or area, use another sweet, fleshy fruit – perhaps a mango chutney from the jar, or raspberry jam with a dash of vinegar or red wine added for that slightly tangy bite.

Prep time: 30 min.
Cook time: 0 min.
Storage time: 1 day in the fridge (if you keep the dressing separate)
Suitable diets: Vegan, Vegetarian, Gluten-Free, Paleo

Calories: 230 kcal
Protein: 5.2 g
Carbs: 27.8 g
Fat: 10.9 g (2 grams of which saturates)
Makes: 4 portions

Ingredients:
- 8 Chinese leaves (or Napa cabbage)
- 1 large carrot
- 1 cucumber
- 6 scallions or spring onions
- 8 slices of dried mango
- ½ cup of cashews

TAMARIND DRESSING
- 2 ounces of tamarind pulp or 1 ½ teaspoons of tamarind paste
- ½ teaspoon Szechuan peppercorns
- 2 teaspoons sesame oil
- 1 garlic clove
- ½ teaspoon brown sugar

- 2 tablespoons cilantro / coriander
- Himalayan salt to taste

Instructions:

To make the dressing: Put the tamarind pulp in a small glass bowl. Add 1 cup of warm water and let it soak for about one quarter of an hour. Then, squeeze the tamarind through your fingers in the water and continue to press or pinch it until it's been mixed nicely into a pulp. Press through a strainer or sieve.

Put 6 tablespoons of the strained tamarind water, the Szechuan pepper, sesame oil, garlic, sugar and chopped herbs into a screw-top jar, shake well, and set aside.

To make the salad: Slice the cabbage or Chinese leaves thinly. Shred or grate the carrot. Cut the cucumber in half, remove the seeds from the center, and slice it very thinly. (The consistency of the salad makes a big difference in your enjoyment of it! The dressing can blend better with the ingredients, I feel.)

Slice the spring onion at a diagonal and chop the dried mango. Chop the cashews if you'd prefer, but I like to keep them whole or halved as something to 'chew on'.

Toss the ingredients together, place onto 4 separate plates, and drizzle the dressing on top to serve.

More-Than-A-Mouthful Sprouted Salad

We came up with this name because the salad is simply so good that we tend to eat it with a large spoon, our youngest fitting too much in his mouth to chew! The texture is divine, and just like bite-sized snacks, they add to the tastiness of the overall experience.

Prep time: 20 min. (plus soaking nuts 6-12 hours)
Cook time: 0 min.
Storage time: 1 day in the fridge (if you keep the dressing separate)
Suitable diets: Vegan, Vegetarian, Gluten-Free, Paleo, Raw, Properly Combined

Calories: 382 kcal
Protein: 17.4 g
Carbs: 51.7 g
Fat: 14.9 g (0.9 grams of which saturates)
Makes: 4 portions

Ingredients:
- ⅔ cup cherry tomatoes
- 4 ounces (or a couple handfuls) of alfalfa sprouts
- 4 ounces (") of lentil sprouts
- 1 handful of fresh, Italian flat-leaf parsley
- 2 cups of fresh baby spinach
- ¾ cup walnuts
- 1 red bell pepper (or 'capsicum')
- 1 ½ cups red cabbage
- 2 carrots
- 2 apples (leave out if you're following a properly combined diet)
- 1 cup of celery
- ¾ cup radishes
- 1 ½ cups beet (or 'beetroot')
- salad dressing of your choice, or a simple balsamic vinegar with olive oil

- salt and pepper to taste

Instructions:

The way you chop the vegetables makes a big difference to the texture of the salad. I prefer thin slices about three-quarters inch long, so they're just small enough to fit in your mouth.

The sprouts are quite easy to make at home. And don't forget to soak the nuts in water overnight or for at least 6 hours, preparing them in the Paleo way for proper absorption of the minerals.

Chop the ingredients, making sure to shred the cabbage. Use spiralizer on the beet if you'd like. Add all the ingredients together in a large bowl, and add as much dressing as desired.

[4.3] Soups & Stews

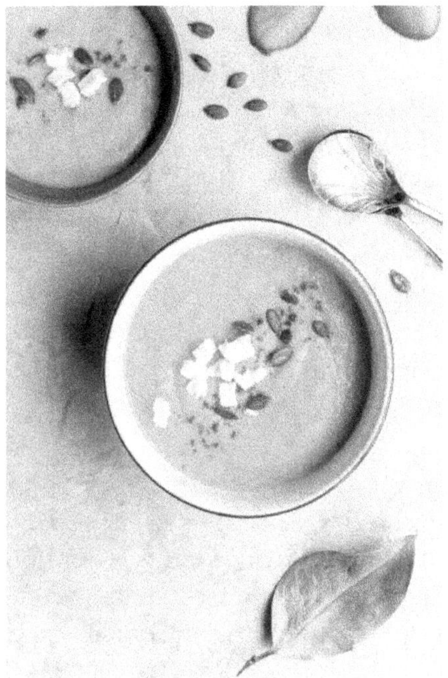

Soups are an absolute must-have in every home, during every season. Here are some reasons why I'm so crazy about liquid meals:

- **All Season:** Even during hot summer days you can drink a cooling gazpacho (cold Spanish tomato soup)
- **Weight Loss:** The warmth and the liquid make you feel more full than the same amount of calories would in a 'standard' meal, for example a sandwich or a casserole. That's why they're great for losing and maintaining weight.
- **Storage:** They freeze really well. The only soups that haven't thawed out and been as good as fresh were ones I experimented with (those recipes are not in this book!) had rice in them. Otherwise, you can freeze any homemade soup for 6 months or maybe even longer.
- **Eliminate Food Waste:** I'm a firm believer in the adage "waste not, want not" and will spare you the rant here in this recipe section. Not only are you saving money by saving food, but you're also helping to save the planet! Soups are a

great way to cook up carrots, celery and other veggies that are going soft. And if potatoes or other tubers are going bad or have spots on them? Simply cut off the bad parts and boil the rest. Unlike a casserole, patatas bravas, or baked potatoes, things in soups generally don't have to look their best – they usually get blended or puréed anyway.

- **Easy to Transport:** If you have a tight seal on your container, you're good to go! I often reuse large glass pickle jars or olive jars to store my soup in the fridge or freezer, and take those jars with me to work or out on a hike. I don't mind parting with the jars if I end up recycling them. It's better than taking my good Tupperware or other storage containers that end up 'wandering off' at work into someone else's home!

- **Meal on the Go:** If you have a Thermos that you haven't put coffee in yet (because the smell lingers and makes your food taste a bit weird), then it's perfect to put a well-blended soup into. It'll stay warm for up to 8 hours in a well-insulated Thermos container, meaning you can heat it up in the morning as you're preparing yourself (and probably the rest of the family) for the day. On your lunch break, do a few yoga asanas or hit the fitness center for a half hour, and sip your soup casually at your desk or on the drive / walk back to work. This isn't a good suggestion if you're trying to eat mindfully… but sometimes there are only so many hours in a day, and we have to choose what we can achieve in what little time we have!

Miso & Sweet Potato Soup

Prep time: 10 min.
Cook time: 40 min.
Storage time: Up to 5 days in the fridge or 5 months in the freezer
Suitable diets: Gluten-Free, Vegan, Vegetarian
Servings: 3 adult-size portions

Calories*: 242 kcal
Protein*: 10.1 g
Carbs*: 33.3 g
Fat*: 6 g (0.7 grams of which saturates)
*Per portion

Ingredients:

- 4 teaspoons of vegetable (or sunflower) oil
- 6 spring onions, finely chopped
- 2 thumb-sized pieces of ginger, finely chopped
- 2 cloves of garlic, finely chopped (or 2 teaspoons if you buy it pre-chopped)
- 2 tablespoons white miso
- 2 medium sweet potatoes, peeled and cut into small pieces
- 750ml* or three pints of vegetable stock
- 2 large handfuls of shredded kale
  I usually use Imperial measurements like cups and ounces, but this size is quite handy for me to recognize and guesstimate… because it's the same amount of liquid that a bottle of wine has!

Instructions:

Heat 2 teaspoons of oil in a large pan. Chop the spring onion / scallion, and add half to the pan. Press the garlic and finely chop the ginger. Add to the pan a sautée for 6-10 minutes, or until soft.

Chop the sweet potatoes into large chunks. Add the sweet potatoes to the pan. Put a lid on the pan and let simmer about 25-30 minutes. You'll know the potatoes are done when you can poke them easily through with a fork.

Add to a blender, or use a stick blender. (You might want to let the mixture cool down a little first.) Add back to the pan and keep warm as you heat 2 teaspoons of oil in a frying pan and fry the remaining spring onions, ginger and garlic over high heat for about 2-3 minutes or until they have softened. Reduce heat, add the chopped kale (mine is usually sold pre-chopped in a bag) and about 3 tablespoons of water, and cook for 2-3 minutes until the kale has wilted. Stir in the miso and salt and pepper to taste. Garnish with a bit more kale and spring onions.

Health-Restoring Chili & Rice Stew

In many Asian countries, boiled rice soups are very popular. In China, they are called *congees* and often consumed in the morning for breakfast. Rice soups and stews have a different, almost acquired taste than we normally know rice to have. This is because it breaks down during boiling and continues to soak up liquid even after having cooled. Rice in these stews is often softer, more inflated, and a kind of viscous white 'porridge' which is simply delicious to enjoy any time of year!

Depending on whether you choose to add more chili, garlic, and ginger into this soup, it's either a wonderful meal to cure the common cold, or it's a powerful expectorant (making your nose run and moving phlegm out of your lungs). Either way, it's a must-have in the freezer for when you feel a cold coming on. I absolutely swear by this stew during the changing of seasons when our body is adjusting to temperature and barometric pressure changes, thereby being more susceptible to catching colds, sniffles, or fevers.

Prep time: 10 min.
Cook time: 40 min.
Storage time: Up to 5 days in the fridge or 5 months in the freezer
Suitable diets: Gluten-Free, Vegan, Vegetarian
Servings: 4 adult-size portions

Calories*: 432 kcal
Protein*: 9.3 g
Carbs*: 69.6 g
Fat*: 12.8 g (1.4 grams of which saturates)
*Per portion

Ingredients:
- 2 tablespoons vegetable or sunflower oil
- 4 teaspoons sesame oil (or walnut if you prefer the flavor)
- 4 garlic cloves, chopped finely or pureed / pressed
- 9 scallions or spring onions, finely chopped
- 4 teaspoons finely grated fresh ginger
- 2 small red chiles, seeds removed and sliced very thinly

- 1 cup long-grain white rice
- 12 cups vegetable soup stock
- 2 tablespoons soy sauce
- 2 bunches of spring greens*, roughly shredded
- 2 small bunches of cilantro / coriander, finely chopped
- ground white pepper to taste

"Spring greens" are sometimes sold in grocery stores with that exact label on the packaging. Otherwise, feel free to use a mix of cabbage, kale, spinach, and lettuce.

Super Saver Tip: Use the leafy green parts of radishes, carrots, tops of celery stalks and more for a simple green 'place holder' in casseroles, soups, and stews like this one. They are indeed edible, though they don't taste as sweet as spinach nor as bitter crisp as kale. Store them in the freezer for up to 4 months if you don't have immediate use for them.

Instructions:

Peel off the rough brown 'skin' of the garlic with a teaspoon. A friend who travels to India frequently taught me that. Using a spoon rather than a knife ensures that less of the actual root is cut off. Ginger peel or 'skin' is edible, but very tough and bitter-tasting, which is why it's removed. Chop the scallions or spring onions finely.

Pour both oils into a medium-sized saucepan and set to high heat. Add the garlic and scallions (or spring onions) and sautée until the garlic has reached a golden brown color and is just starting to burn.

Add the ginger, chile and rice to the saucepan. Stir-fry the mixture like this for 1 minute, then add the soy sauce and soup stock. Wait a few minutes until the mixture has been brought to a boil, then cover the saucepan with a lid and turn the heat down to a low setting. Leave for 30 minutes, stirring occasionally.

Add the spring greens, keeping the heat low, and cover. Let cook for another 5 minutes maximum, depending on how soft or *al dente* (crunchy or chewy) you'd like your greens to be.

Serve with coriander / cilantro sprinkled on top with pinches of white pepper. Or, ladle directly into freezer-safe containers and let cool completely before putting into your freezer.

Tip If Cooking For Children: If you let the soup sit in your fridge for a few days, the spicy heat of the soup grows in intensity. If it's too hot for your palate (often, children don't like spicy foods), then simply add more pre-boiled rice or potatoes to thin out the spice.

Nutritional Tip: Remember, the more you cook vegetables, the more you lose vital nutrients in the food. Vitamins are more fragile than minerals. Vitamin C especially is very susceptible to being damaged from light (letting lettuce sit in the sun, for example), air (think of apples going brown), and heat (cooking, baking, other heat sources like oranges sitting in a hot car).

Spicy, Smoked Bean Stew

Remember to **soak the beans overnight** in order to soften them up for good cooking. (Or if you're on a Paleo diet, soak them longer to just start them growing.)

Prep time: 12 hours (soaking beans) plus 15 min.
Cook time: 1 hour 20 min.
Storage time: Up to 7 days in the fridge or 6 months in the freezer
Suitable diets: Gluten-Free, Vegan, Vegetarian, Paleo
Servings: 4 adult-size portions

Calories*: 198 kcal
Protein*: 4.3 g
Carbs*: 30.3 g
Fat*: 8.6 g (2.1 grams of which saturates)
*Per portion

Ingredients:

- ½ cup dried great northern beans or butter beans or lima beans
- 2 tablespoons olive oil
- 1 large onion
- 2 garlic cloves
- 2 teaspoons *pimentón dulce* (Spanish or Moroccan smoked sweet paprika)
- 1 celery stick / stalk
- 1 carrot
- 2 medium potatoes
- 1 red bell pepper (or "capsicum")
- 2 cups of veggie stock or 3 cubes of vegetable stock
- Himalaya salt and ground black pepper to taste

Instructions:

Soak the beans overnight. Drain the water and place them into a large saucepan. Re-fill with just enough water to cover them, and bring to a boil. Reduce heat and let cook on medium heat for about 30 minutes, or until they've softened.

Chop the onion, press the garlic, then slice the celery, carrots, potatoes and bell pepper.

Put the oil into a different saucepan, bring to a medium heat, then add the onion. Sautée for 4-5 minutes or until softened and translucent. Add the garlic and pimentón, cooking for another 2 minutes. Add celery, carrots, potatoes, red bell pepper and cook for 2 minutes, stirring constantly to coat the vegetables in oil.

Add the vegetable stock (or water, with the cubes sprinkled into the pan by crushing them with your fingers) and beans, and bring to a boil. Reduce the heat immediately and cover most of the pan with a lid. Let simmer for 40 minutes on low heat. Stir often to ensure all vegetables are cooked.

Season to taste with salt and pepper. Serve with bread if you'd like, or a dash of paprika powder on top for added color.

Moroccan-Style Lentil Stew

This stew, as with many dishes from Northern Africa and the Middle East, is often served with warm pita bread. It helps soak up the last delicious drops of the stew.

<u>Remember to soak the lentils in water overnight!</u>

Prep time: 10 min.

Cook time: 45 min.

Storage time: Up to 10 days in the fridge or 8 months in the freezer

Suitable diets: Gluten-Free, Vegan, Vegetarian

Servings: 4 adult-size portions

Calories*: 310 kcal

Protein*: 14.1 g

Carbs*: 52.3 g

Fat*: 5.8 g (0.4 grams of which saturates)

*Per portion

Ingredients:

- ¾ cup dried lentils (any color you'd like, whether brown or red etc.)
- 1 small red onion
- 1 yellow bell pepper (also called "capsicum")
- 2 tablespoons tomato purée or paste
- 2 teaspoons sweet smoked paprika (if you can't find any, use smoked garlic instead if you'd like)
- 1 teaspoon ground cumin
- ½ teaspoon ground coriander
- 2 garlic cloves, finely chopped (or *only* 2 teaspoons of smoked garlic – you don't need to ward off any vampires, so don't overdo it with the garlic)
- 2x 14-ounce cans of chopped tomatoes
- 1 large handful of fresh baby spinach or ½ cup of frozen spinach
- 1 tablespoon of tahini sesame paste
- 1 tablespoon of agave syrup, coconut flower syrup, or honey (if you're not strictly vegan)
- ½ bunch or 2 handfuls of chopped parsley, to serve

- toasted or warmed pita bread, to serve
- pinch of saffron, to serve
- pinch of salt or Bragg's Amino Acids, to taste
- enough vegetable oil or olive for frying

Soak the lentils in unsalted water overnight. Just as a quick note: potatoes and pasta are often boiled in water with a pinch or two of salt added. If you boil beans, lentils, and other legumes with salt then they will become too chewy in consistency.

Put the lentils in a medium-sized saucepan with 3 cups of water. Bring to a boil, then turn down the heat to a medium-low gas mark 2 or 3. Cover with a lid and let cook for 17-20 minutes. Ideally, they'll be a bit *al dente* or slightly undercooked. (It's hard to describe that word, being an Italian!) The reason is that you'll cook the lentils a bit more later on. So you don't want them turning into mush at the end!

While the lentils are cooking, heat a small amount of oil on medium heat in a large frying pan or skillet. Choose one that has high sides and preferably also a lid. Add the chopped onion and bell pepper, season to taste with salt and pepper, and sauté for 4-6 minutes or until the onion has become translucent / clear, but not brown on the edges. You want it soft, not burnt.

Stir in the tomato purée or paste, and cook for another minute. Add the rest of the spices (including the garlic) and cook for another half minute. Stir in the chopped tomatoes – do not drain the liquid from the can before adding them. Cover the pan with a lid if you have one (because it will keep more of the spice flavor in) and simmer over low heat for 15 minutes.

By the time you've finished the tomato mixing and simmering, and have cleaned up the kitchen a bit, the lentils should be ready. Drain the excess water from the pan, and add the lentils. Cook for another 10 minutes without the lid, so the liquid can escape in steam form. This makes the stew a bit more solid and hearty.

Turn off the heat and stir in the spinach. Remember, you don't want to over-cook vegetables, because you'll lose much of the nutrients in them. The spinach will 'wilt' or half-cook with the heat of the stew. Stir in the agave syrup or honey, or whichever sweetener you've chosen that will offset the acidity of the tomatoes. Serve with chopped parsley sprinkled atop.

Low-Cal Vegetable Soup

Prep time: 15 min.
Cook time: 20 min.
Storage time: Up to 7 days in the fridge or 3 months in the freezer
Suitable diets: Gluten-Free, Vegan, Vegetarian, Paleo
Servings: 6 adult-size portions

Calories*: 67 kcal
Protein*: 3.5 g
Carbs*: 10.1 g
Fat*: 1.6 g (0.3 grams of which saturates)
*Per portion

Ingredients:

- 2 teaspoons of olive oil
- 1 medium-sized onion
- 2 garlic cloves
- 2 stalks of celery
- 2 carrots
- 1 can of chopped tomatoes (usually 12 or 16 ounces)
- 2 tablespoons tomato paste or purée
- 2 cubes of vegetable stock
- 3 pints of water*
- 2 medium zucchinis (also called "courgettes")
- ¾ cup green beans
- ½ cup frozen peas
- Himalayan salt and ground black pepper to taste
  This is the equivalent of filling the tomato can about 3-4 times with water, then pouring it into the soup pot. It's a great way to make sure you're using all the little pieces of tomato that could be stuck to the bottom of the can.

Instructions:

Heat the oil in a large saucepan and fry the onion, garlic, carrots, and finely sliced celery in it. I usually 'string' the celery first, pulling off the long vertical strings of darker green color that tend to make it a bit more bitter and chewy tasting. At least, it's an old habit left over from my mother!

After frying for 5 minutes, add the chopped tomatoes and tomato purée or paste. Crumble up the veggie stock cubes in your fingers while adding it to the pot. Mix well, then add the water. Bring to a boil, then reduce heat and let cook for another 5 minutes. Stir occasionally.

Add the chopped zucchini, chopped green beans and peas (straight from the freezer into the pot) and simmer for another 5-7 minutes. The vegetables should be tender but still *al dente*, firm enough to chew. This ensures much of the nutrients remain. Season the soup with salt and pepper.

Variations:

In the fall I love to 'spice up' this soup with 2 more cloves of garlic and 1 tablespoon of cayenne pepper. I also use chili-infused olive oil. I feel the extra spice staves off colds, and helps warm up your body while the weather is growing colder! I also think that I eat smaller portions when there's a lot of spices, so it helps me grow accustomed to eating smaller portions (some call it 'shrinking the stomach' naturally) and losing a couple pounds over a few weeks this way.

Lemongrass Pumpkin Soup

If you don't have the fresh root ingredients listed here on hand, a good rule of thumb is to substitute 1 unit of the fresh root or herb with ⅔ of the dried variation. Make sure to leave plenty of time for the dried herbs to moisten into the oil, soup stock or other liquid to release their flavor.

This soup freezes very well, and is a fast and easy favorite to grab when working late and in need of a quick family pleaser.

Prep time: 15 min.
Cook time: 18 min.
Storage time: Up to 5 days in the fridge or 3 months in the freezer
Suitable diets: Gluten-Free, Vegan, Vegetarian, Paleo
Servings: 4 adult-size portions

Calories*: 383 kcal
Protein*: 8.9 g
Carbs*: 56.1 g
Fat*: 18.6 g (16.1 grams of which saturates)
*Per portion

Ingredients:
- 2 brown onions
- 2 lemongrass stalks
- 2 long red (hot) chilis
- ½ bunch or roughly 1 cup of coriander
- 2-inch piece of fresh galangal or ginger root
- 2-inch piece of turmeric
- 2 garlic cloves
- zest or peel of ½ lime
- 2 quarts of vegetable stock OR 8 cubes mixed with 6 cups (=2 quarts) of water
- 1 cup of coconut cream

- 8 kaffir lime leaves or a dash of lime juice (optional)
- 1 1/3 tablespoons coconut oil
- 2 medium-sized pumpkins, seeds and stringy parts removed

<u>Food Saver Tip</u>: After digging the seeds out with a spoon, keep them. Wipe of the stringy parts or any flesh on them, and lay flat on a baking tray. Bake at 400-425°F on the top tray for about 10 minutes or until they're dried out and much lighter in color. Dust with salt or your own spicy seasoning as a great, protein-packed snack.

Instructions:

Dice the onions. Separate the coriander stems / stalks and the leaves. Chop the leaves (or leave them whole for pretty looking garnish). Chop the coriander stems / stalks and the lemon grass into roughly 3-inch pieces. (They'll just be thrown into the blender later anyway.)

Sauté the onion, lemongrass, coriander stalks, chili, galangal (or ginger), tumeric and lime leaves in the coconut oil in a large soup pot on medium heat for 2-3 minutes or until they've all softened slightly.

Chop up the pumpkin into small cubes. Throw it into the pot with pressed / crushed garlic, lime zest (also called 'peel') and veggie soup stock. Bring to a boil, then turn down the heat and simmer for 15 minutes, adding the coconut cream. Keep a bit of the coconut cream for serving, as the color looks splendid on top of the bright orange soup. Cover the pot with a lid to keep the flavor and the heat in. Check that the pumpkin has become soft by poking it with a fork.

Remove the lime peel, lime leaves (if you've used them) and lemongrass from the soup. They will remain tough and chewy, which is what you don't want in a smooth and creamy soup! The flavor has been transferred to the soup during cooking, so it's okay to discard or compost these now.

Transfer the soup to a blender, or blend it well with a stick mixer. Purée until smooth. Add the remaining small amount of coconut cream on top, adding the coriander leaves on top as well. (Skip the sprinkling of fresh herbs if you'll freeze the soup in batches.)

[4.4] Pasta

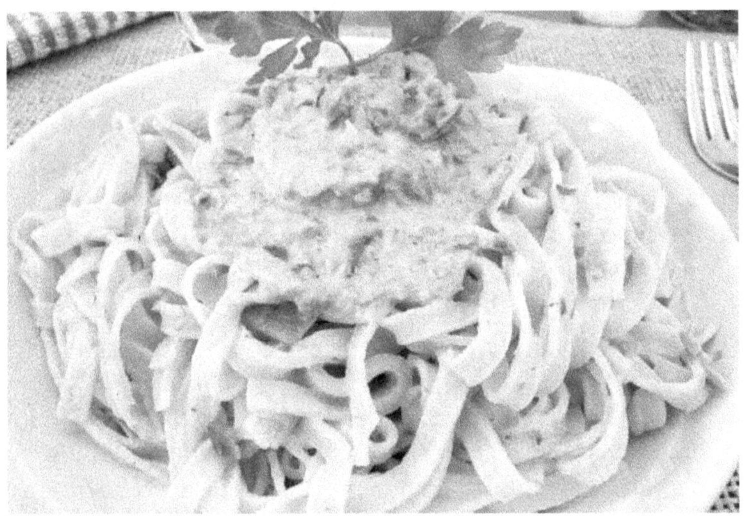

Savory Mushroom Pasta with Artichoke Sage Sauce

Leeks are used in this sauce, and are used to add a very mild taste reminiscent of cabbage. They look essentially like really large spring onions (or 'scallions'), being about as wide in circumference as the space between your thumb and index finger if you were to make a circle of them (the 'A-OK' sign with the other three fingers extended). If you cannot find leeks, I suggest using iceberg lettuce as a water kind of placeholder to thin out the sauce a bit and sneak some extra vegetables into your meal.

Prep time: 15 min.
Cook time: 18 min.
Storage time: Up to 5 days in the fridge or 3 months in the freezer
Suitable diets: Gluten-Free, Vegan, Vegetarian, Paleo
Servings: 4 adult-size portions

Calories*: 440 kcal

Protein*: 17.5 g
Carbs*: 69.7 g
Fat*: 11.9 g (1.4 grams of which saturates)
*Per portion

Ingredients:
- 1 pound dry pasta (tagliatelle, fettuccine, linguine, or spaghetti)
- 1 pound sliced mushrooms
- 2 leeks
- 8 teaspoons extra virgin olive oil
- salt and pepper to taste

Artichoke Sauce:
- 2 jars of artichoke hearts (about 3 cups when drained)
- ½ cup olive oil
- 20 fresh sage leaves (or take about 2 teaspoons dry, soaking them for 4+ hours in a couple tablespoons of water to soften)
- 4 garlic cloves
- 1 teaspoon each of Himalaya salt and freshly ground green or black pepper
- splash of lemon to taste
- grated cheese (see our nut cheese recipe later in this chapter) to serve

Instructions:
Preheat the oven to 400°F / Gas Mark 6.

Wash and slice the leeks (or lettuce if you're using that instead) and toss in a large bowl with half (4 tablespoons) olive oil along with a sprinkling of salt and pepper to taste. Place on waxed baking paper on a baking sheet. Put in the oven and roast for 5 minutes or until they're just turning dark brown on the edges but not burnt.

Bring a large pot of salted water to a boil, then add the pasta. Cook to *al dente*.

While the water is boiling, heat 4 tablespoons of olive oil in a large skillet over medium heat, sautéeing the mushrooms. Season with salt and pepper to taste, then set aside.

Now, make the Artichoke sauce: Drain the artichoke hearts and place them in a blender or mash them very well by hand if you have a solid, sturdy potato masher. Add one cup of lukewarm water, the olive oil, sage, garlic, salt and pepper. Blend in a blender or with a stick blender until creamy and very smooth. Add a splash of lemon juice if you'd like.

Add the leeks from the oven back into the large bowl they were in. Add the cooked, drained pasta (do not rinse) into the bowl. Add the sautéed mixture from the frying pan, and toss vigorously. Add salt and pepper to taste, serving at room temperature or chilled with a bit of grated cheese (optionally) to taste.

Homemade Orecchiette From Scratch

Orecchiette is very similar in shape to gnocchi. It's a tasty, bite-size little dough ball made of wheat flour (whereas gnocchi is made with a mixture of wheat and potato flour). The word 'Orecchiette' literally means 'small (cute) ears' in Italian, and is a specialty of Puglia in south-east Italy.

You don't need a pasta machine to make orecchiette. They're a super fun, hands-on activity when you're entertaining dinner guests – and a delightful activity for children to be involved in, too! **Freeze them uncooked** and pop them into boiling water (without thawing) when you're ready to enjoy.

Prep time: 20 min.
Cook time: 5 min.
Storage time: Up to 2 days in the fridge or 3 months in the freezer
Suitable diets: Vegan, Vegetarian
Servings: 4 adult-size portions

Calories*: 430 kcal
Protein*: 10.5 g
Carbs*: 77.5 g
Fat*: 8 g (1.2 grams of which saturates)
*Per portion

Ingredients:
- 3 ¼ cups white flour (plus extra for dusting)
- 2 tablespoons extra virgin olive oil
- ½ teaspoon finely ground Himalaya salt

Instructions:
Put all of the flour into a large bowl. Make a well in the center and pour in the oil and 9.5 fluid ounces of warm water. (That's about one cup plus a small splash extra.) Sprinkle the salt over everything in the bowl.

Use the handle of a wooden spoon to mix the flour into the liquid gradually. Once it's mixed well enough, feel free to use the spoon as you normally would to mix the rest, scraping the flour off the bottom and edges of the bowl to combine with the rest of the dough. The resulting texture should be crumbly like breadcrumbs.

Turn out the mixture onto a well-floured surface (like your counter top or dining room table). Knead the mixture until you have a soft, smooth dough – this should take about 8 minutes. If you've never kneaded dough by hand before, don't worry! It involves a lot more muscle than you'd expect, but is fun to do: Hold the dough in one hand while you use the other hand to fold the rest over on top of the ball you have (kind of piling it on top), pushing it down while stretching / pulling the dough away from the other hand. Make sure to rotate the dough about 45° (or just about two "hours" on a clock) as you go.

Divide the dough into pieces and roll them between the palms of your hands, so you've got several long 'ropes' or 'snakes' of dough. They should each be about the same thickness as your pinkie (smallest) finger.

Cut the 'ropes' with a knife into small pieces approximately ½ inch in length, or about the same length as your thumbnail. Dust them with flour.

Place the dough on a floured surface and press into them with your thumb to shape the 'little ears' Place them on a floured baking tray or other flat surface until you are ready to cook them. Alternatively, you can freeze them in flat layers very well for up to 3 months.

Cook the orecchiette in a large pan of boiling water (don't forget to add a pinch of salt to the water as it's being brought to a boil!) for about 5 minutes. **<u>You know they are ready when they float up to the surface</u>**, just like the way gnocchi cook. Do not rinse before serving. Add the sauce and other parts of the dish immediately (I keep them warm on the stovetop) and add a bit of ground pepper to taste.

Variations:

You can be creative in how you serve this delicious and easy to make pasta.

- With green pesto, olive oil, and fresh basil leaves

- With red pesto, olive oil, sun-dried tomatoes, and a sprinkling of dried chili flakes
- With bolognese / red pasta sauce and chunks of fried tofu, 'fake' tofu meatballs or other vegetable-based meat replacements
- With spicy roasted vegetables and a drizzling of olive oil (see next recipe)

Roasted Vegetables with Orecchiette Pasta and Wine-Infused Onion

This dish is a quick and easy family favorite that's easy to reheat in the oven for leftovers the next day. Oddly enough, I wouldn't recommend storing the leftovers in the refrigerator. The cold makes the water and oil separate more from the vegetables, which in turn 'drown' the pasta ever so slightly. If you haven't licked your fingers then placed them into the food, this will stay just fine for 24-48 hours in an airtight or covered container. Bacteria, mold and other things start growing in more moist, humid and warmer climates.

As you grow more comfortable with veggies and cooking, feel free to substitute any of these vegetables for other ones, or add more!

Prep time: 20-25 min.
Cook time: 40 min.
Storage time: Up to 1 days in an airtight container
Suitable diets: Vegan, Vegetarian
Servings: 4 adult-size portions

Calories*: 498 kcal
Protein*: 9.8 g
Carbs*: 56.3 g
Fat*: 27 g (3.7 grams of which saturates)
*Per portion

Ingredients:
- 1 large red onion
- 1 small eggplant
- 1 large zucchini
- 2 yellow bell peppers (or 'capsicum')
- 1 medium-sized head of broccoli
- 2 teaspoons dried chili flakes
- 2 tablespoons fresh rosemary leaves
- ½ cup extra virgin olive oil
- 1 glass (about 4-5 ounces) dry white wine
- 1 batch of freshly made orecchiette (see previous recipe)

- Salt to taste
- Pecorino or parmesan cheese to grate on top, if you're not following a vegan diet

Instructions:

Preheat the oven to 400°F or gas mark 6. Cut the onion into 12 large chunks. Cut the bell pepper(removing its stems and seeds), zucchini, and eggplant into large yet manageable chunks (about 1" square, each).

Place the onion, pepper, zucchini and eggplant into a medium sized bowl. Sprinkle over the chili flakes, rosemary, and salt. Then drizzle over two-thirds of the oil. Stir well with your hands until the mixture is evenly coated. Pour out onto a baking dish.

Roast the vegetables for 15 minutes. Meanwhile, cut the broccoli. (I usually save the large, thick stems in the freezer to add to soups or smoothies. They're quite large and chewy, without much flavor, but still edible! Food waste can be completely eliminated if we're creative and plan ahead well!)

After the veggies have been roasting for 15 minutes, add the broccoli and remaining oil to the pan of vegetables, stirring well with a spoon to ensure they're coated evenly. Let them roast for another 10 minutes.

Cook your homemade orecchiette (this takes about 5 minutes) or a different type of 'chunky' pre-made pasta such as penne or farfalle (bow-tie). While that's boiling, turn off the oven and drizzle the white wine atop the vegetables. (If you have young children sharing this meal, you may want to leave out the chili flakes and substitute 1/3 the amount of vinegar for the wine – or simply bake the wine right from the start, which will cook off all the alcohol content.)

Leave the vegetables and wine mixture in the oven with the door closed or open just a crack, so they stay warm but no longer continue to cook. When the pasta is finished, add it to the tray, toss, and serve with pepper (or grated cheese) to taste.

Spaghetti with Red Sauce from Scratch

This dish is amazingly easy to throw together. The sauce can be stored very well in the fridge or freezer for a long time, which is why I use it as a staple for a quick, throw-together meal along with tofu, 'fake' meatball, butternut squash, or another placeholder to put on top of spaghetti.

Prep time: 5 min.
Cook time: 20 min.
Storage time: Up to 10 days in the refrigerator or 5 months in the freezer
Suitable diets: Vegan, Vegetarian, Paleo*, Gluten-Free*
Servings: 4 adult-size portions
*Most grocery stores carry gluten-free spaghetti. You can make your own using gluten-free flour. Or for a Paleo diet, combine the sauce with any other staple such as roasted potato, butternut squash, rice or homemade paleo onion bread (see the recipe in the earlier chapter).

Calories*: 559 kcal
Protein*: 13.4 g
Carbs*: 74.1 g
Fat*: 24.2 g (3.5 grams of which saturates)
*Per portion

Ingredients:
- 6 tablespoons extra virgin olive oil
- 3 garlic cloves
- 2 tablespoons capers
- 1 medium-sized hot chili (or if you can't find fresh, use 1 ½ teaspoons dried flakes, pre-soaked in water for 10 min.)
- 15 Kalamata olives (pitted, of course – or chopped if you're buying from a can)
- 2 cans of chopped tomatoes
- 1 teaspoon of dried oregano
- ¾ pound of dried spaghetti*
  *My rule of thumb is that a portion of dried pasta the size of your fist is enough for one adult-sized portion when cooked. So if using

macaroni, the amount of macaroni fitting into your hands when they're cupped together — not brimming or overflowing — is the perfect amount for one adult-sized portion.

Instructions:

Heat the oil in a large frying pan over medium heat. Chop the garlic finely (or press it if you have a garlic press) and add it to the pan. Chop the olives into quarters, if you haven't already bought a can of chopped olives. Drain the water from the can of capers.

As soon as the garlic starts to sizzle in the pan, add the capers, chili and olives. Fry for about half a minute.

Stir in the two cans of tomatoes and oregano. Gently simmer on medium-low heat, uncovered, for about 15 minutes. Stir occasionally as you cook the pasta.

Pour the water out of the boiled pasta — I use a strainer / sieve / colander or simply hold the lid close to the edge as I pour out the water, so no pasta slips through into the sink. Put the pasta back into the pot it was cooking in, add the sauce, and put it back onto the stovetop. Stir for about 30 seconds, then turn off the stove and add the pasta with sauce to pre-heated serving dishes. Sprinkle freshly ground pepper on top to serve.

Spaghetti with Artichoke White Wine Sauce

Again, as with the recipe above, feel free to substitute one-third the amount of white wine called for in this recipe with white wine vinegar or apple cider vinegar. You might prefer the more acidic taste of vinegar, or want to play it safe if you're feeding children and pregnant women.

<u>Speaking of wine substitutes…</u> This is a shameless plug, I'm sorry! But if it helps just one or two people reading this, then it's worth it! Alcoholism is a subject still shrouded in shame and guilt, and therefore not discussed much among friends and family. Due to my own personal experiences knowing people suffering from alcoholism and addictions, I've experimented with many ways to enjoy food and beverages without alcohol in them. (See the non-alcoholic 'Ginger Beer' recipe in the next sub-chapter.)

In fact, the first book I wrote and published on Amazon Kindle is about overcoming and dealing with alcoholism. It covers the wide spectrum of support groups, natural healing methods available, and more. Please look up my name "Silvia Pala" on your Kindle, and you'll see that book too. It is available at the following link https://www.amazon.com/dp/B07ZJJ2X3R/. I'd be very grateful if you could leave me some feedback in the review section. My goal is to make our collective lives more enriched, healthy and peaceful – and so your feedback is crucial in knowing I'm on the right track!

Prep time: 15 min.
Cook time: 20 min.
Storage time: Up to 10 days in the refrigerator or 5 months in the freezer
Suitable diets: Vegan, Vegetarian, Paleo*, Gluten-Free*
Servings: 4 adult-size portions
*Most grocery stores carry gluten-free spaghetti. You can make your own using gluten-free flour. Or for a Paleo diet, combine the sauce with any other staple such as roasted potato, butternut squash, rice or homemade paleo onion bread (see the recipe in the earlier chapter).

Calories*: 742 kcal
Protein*: 18.6 g
Carbs*: 78.1 g

Fat*: 29.7 g (4.4 grams of which saturates)
*Per portion

Ingredients:
- 8 tablespoons olive oil (feel free to re-use the oil from the artichokes' jar)
- 12 artichoke hearts (I usually get these in a glass jar)
- 2 red onions
- 3 tablespoons chopped fresh rosemary
- 2 cups frozen peas (thaw them out before cooking with them)
- 1 small head of radicchio (or rocket)
- 1 very small glass (about 3 ounces) of white wine
- ¾ pound of dried spaghetti
- salt and pepper to taste

Instructions:

Heat the oil in a large frying pan over medium heat. Chop the onions finely and the rosemary, too. Add to the frying pan and fry gently for about 10 minutes, stirring occasionally. The onions should turn somewhat translucent and soften considerably, but not get brown on the edges.

Add the artichokes, thawed peas and radicchio. (If you're using rocket instead, add that last – you don't want to cook out all the flavor and eat wilted salad!) Fry together for another 5 minutes, while you cook the spaghetti in a separate pot.

Drain the water from the *al dente* (somewhat firm) spaghetti, putting it back in the pot to stay warm. Add an extra tablespoon or so of oil so it doesn't burn. (I have an electric stovetop, so when I've turned off the heat, the burner still stays warm for quite some time.)

Then add the white wine to the sauce and stir for about one minute. Add the vegetable mixture to the spaghetti and stir for about 30 seconds, until it's well combined. Divide the pasta between 4 pre-warmed serving dishes and enjoy with freshly ground pepper to taste.

Paleo-Friendly Veghetti with Homemade Garlic Pine Nut Pesto

If you're up to a hard-core, plant-based diet, then you'll inevitably incorporate quite a few Paleo dishes into your routine. (See an earlier chapter in this book explaining what a Paleolithic diet does and doesn't include.)

Even though this recipe is in the 'pasta' section, I thought I'd include it. There are so many delicious veggie recipes coming up, I had a hard time figuring out how to narrow them down!

I'll admit that for me, being Italian, it was very weird to get used to 'pasta' or 'spaghetti' made from vegetables rather than wheat flour. Some older generations in my family still cannot wrap their head around it! If you find a vegetable spiralizer or 'veggie pasta maker', this stuff is easy to crank out and boil in a matter of minutes, and makes for a lovely base for any sauce or toppings. If you don't have a spiralizer, then simply julienne the vegetables (which means slicing them in long, thin strips).

Prep time: 7 min.
Cook time: 10 min.
Storage time: Up to 2 days in an airtight container
Suitable diets: Vegan, Vegetarian, Paleo, Gluten-Free
Servings: 2 adult-size portions

Calories*: 258 kcal
Protein*: 4.6 g
Carbs*: 13.7 g
Fat*: 22.7 g (3.3 grams of which saturates)
*Per portion

Ingredients:
- 2 zucchinis
- 2 medium-sized carrots
- 1 tablespoon olive oil for frying the 'veghetti'

FOR THE PINE NUT PESTO

- 2-3 tablespoons extra virgin olive oil
- 2 large handfuls of fresh basil
- 1 garlic clove
- 2 tablespoons fermented tofu (optional)
- 1 handful of pine nuts
- 2 teaspoons lemon juice
- Himalayan salt and ground pepper to taste

Instructions:

Place all the pesto ingredients (yes, even the raw garlic) into a blender or food processor and mix well. Add more olive oil if you'd like, until you reach your desired consistency of smooth creaminess.

Heat the one tablespoon of olive oil in a pan over medium heat. Add the spiralized zucchini and carrot, stirring often for 2-3 minutes or until they've soften.

Add the pesto and stir well for 3 minutes.

Add more pine nuts, fresh basil and ground pepper on top to serve.

[4.5] Vegetables

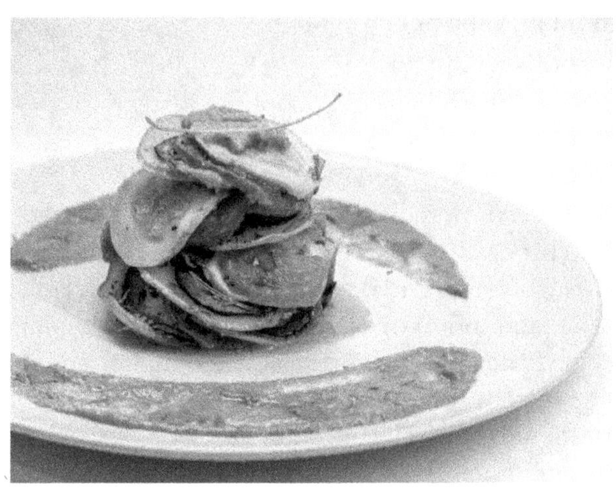

Ratatouille

Prep time: 15 min.

Cook time: 1 hour

Storage time: Up to 2 days in an airtight container (freezing works well, but changes the texture slightly; refrigeration makes the water / moisture separate more from the mixture, changing the texture even more – which is why it's best to simply cover and let sit at room temperature for storage)

Suitable diets: Gluten-Free, Vegan, Vegetarian, Paleo

Servings: 6

Calories*: 147 kcal

Protein*: 2.5 g

Carbs*: 15.1 g

Fat*: 9.7 g (1.4 grams of which saturates)

*Per portion

Ingredients:

- 8 baby eggplants or 2 medium eggplants
- 2 red or yellow bell peppers / capsicums

- 4 medium tomatoes
- 4 zucchini / courgettes
- 2 onions (red, white, or yellow)
- 24–28 garlic cloves (or 4 tablespoons of pre-minced garlic)
- 4–6 tablespoons of fresh herbs, such as thyme or rosemary
- extra virgin olive oil for drizzling
- salt and pepper to taste
- splash of white wine or balsamic vinegar to taste

Instructions:

Preheat the oven to 400° F / Gas Mark 6 and place a piece of wax baking paper on a large baking sheet. (Use two pans if necessary.)

If you're using baby eggplant, slice them in half lengthwise. Or, chop the full-size eggplant into roughly 1" bite-size pieces. Thickly slice the bell pepper / capsicum into inch-wide strips, then cut in half. Cut the tomatoes into large chunks (roughly 6 chunks per tomato). Slice the zucchini the long way and then chop into 1/2 inch thick pieces. Likewise slice the onion in half, then into approximately half-inch thick half moons.

Spread out the veggies on the baking sheet in a single layer, so none are piled up. Add the garlic gloves, unpressed or unchopped – but do remember to peel them! Sprinkle the herbs atop.

Drizzle about ½ cup olive oil over the top and tilt the baking tray from side to side, ensuring the bottoms of all the veggies are well coated. The tops are still raw and not coated in oil, which gives them a lovely crisp texture when roasting.

Roast for about 25 minutes, then flip the mixture with a spatula and roast for another 10-15 minutes, or until the sides now facing up have been cooked visibly.

Turn down the heat to about 275-300°F and roast for another 15-20 minutes, or until the veggie mixture has become tender and the edges begin to caramelize (look golden brown, and taste sweet – you'll know that taste and smell!).

Add salt and pepper to taste, and serve immediately when hot. It serves very well with pasta, polenta, rice, in soft shell tortillas, or on a bed of fresh spring greens.

Peanut Coconut Curry with Eggplant & Zucchini

Prep time: 10 min.
Cook time: 30 min.
Storage time: Up to 5 days in the fridge or 3 months in the freezer
Suitable diets: Gluten-Free, Vegan, Vegetarian, Paleo
Servings: 4

Calories*: 251 kcal
Protein*: 5.5 g
Carbs*: 17 g
Fat*: 15.5 g (7.2 grams of which saturates)
*Per portion

Ingredients:

- 2-5 tablespoons oil for frying (use olive or coconut)
- 1 eggplant
- 1 zucchini
- 2 onions (yellow or white)
- 2 garlic cloves
- 1 piece ginger about the size of your index finger, or 1 heaping tablespoon dried/powdered
- 1 teaspoon cumin seeds
- 1 teaspoon of coriander seeds (crush them a bit to release their flavor)
- 1 teaspoon turmeric
- ½ teaspoon chilli powder
- 1 can of coconut milk
- 1 tablespoon tamarind paste
- 1 tablespoon peanut butter
- freshly chopped coriander to serve
- bread or rice to serve

Instructions:

Heat 1 tablespoon oil in a pan. Cook the eggplant / aubergine in batches until golden and soft, frying it for about 3-5 minutes per batch. Add a bit more oil as you go, if you need to. If you can fry the eggplant all at once, that's even better, but I don't have such a large frying pans and woks don't really cook the same way; hence why I do this in batches.

Take a medium-sized soup pot. Dice the onion and add it to the pot with 1-2 tablespoons of oil and cook until soft and golden, somewhat translucent. Add the finely chopped garlic and ginger, and cook for a minute. Add the spices and cook for 2 more minutes.

Pour in the coconut milk, tamarind paste (or simply use fresh with a couple tablespoons of warm water) and peanut butter. Simmer gently for about 2 minutes or until the peanut butter dissolves.

Add the cooked eggplant back into the pot and simmer for 15 minutes. Turn off the heat, stir through some finely chopped cilantro / coriander and serve with bread or rice.

Stuffed Portobello Mushrooms with Walnut & Thyme

This is a savory, mouth-watering recipe for anyone who likes mushrooms and a more 'meaty' taste – as opposed to a sweet pineapple curry, for example. These mushrooms freeze very well and should be served hot, because cold mushrooms take on a chewier texture that can be mildly unappetizing.

You can eat the stuffed mushrooms as they are, or on top of a burger bun / brioche / coriander bread (the recipe for which is also in this book). I like to serve mine on a bed of baby spinach, leafy greens, and arugula / rocket.

Prep time: 15 min.
Cook time: 18 min.
Storage time: Up to 3 days in the fridge or 2 months in the freezer
Suitable diets: Gluten-Free, Vegan, Vegetarian, Paleo, Low-Sugar
Servings: 2 adult-sized portions

Calories*: 306 kcal
Protein*: 11.4 g
Carbs*: 19.4 g
Fat*: 18.8 g (2.2 grams of which saturates)
*Per portion

Ingredients:
- 4 portobello mushrooms 4 very large, stalks removed and chopped
- 4 tablespoons olive oil (or olive oil cooking spray)
- 1 yellow or red onion
- ¾ cup mushrooms (any kind)
- 1 garlic clove
- 1 teaspoon smoked paprika
- 1 teaspoon fresh thyme leaves
- 1 piece of day-old sourdough bread, crumbled into breadcrumbs, or use a handful of pine nuts or a scant handful of hard tofu, crumbled

- ⅔ cup walnuts

Instructions:

Heat the grill to medium. Cut the large stalks or stems off the portobello mushrooms. Set aside to use later. Spray or sprinkle the portobello mushrooms with some frying oil on both sides, sprinkling on some seasoning, and then and grill for about 3 minutes on high heat, then flip them over and grill the other side. If you don't have a grill or tabletop grill (like the George Foreman brand) then you can alternatively fry it in a pan.

Meanwhile, chop the onion finely. Chop the mushrooms, including the portobello stems. Chop the walnuts and put them in a small pan on medium-low heat to toast. Crush or press the garlic clove.

Take a frying pan, turn on medium heat, and put in 2 tablespoons olive oil with the onion. Sautée until translucent and soft. Add the chopped up mushrooms - this includes the portobello mushroom stalks you've chopped up - and a bit of salt. Sautée until the mushroom mixture is a light golden brownish black.

Add the pressed garlic, smoked paprika and thyme. Stir for a minute, then stir in the breadcrumbs (or the tofu / pine nut alternatives) and walnuts. Stir for 1 minute.

Spoon the mix into the middles of the portobello mushrooms and pack down to fill the cavities. Grill again, for another 5 minutes.

Serve hot with roasted vegetables, steamed / baked potatoes, or on a bed of lettuce. Sprinkle nut cheese (see our other recipe) atop to serve if you're like.

Green Beans with Lemon Toasted Almonds

With simple recipes like these, that have few ingredients, it's important to have high-quality, fresh ingredients. You can use lemon juice from the bottle, of course, but using frozen green beans for this one just doesn't pack the same mouth-watering flavor as their fresh counterparts.

For the almonds – especially if you're Paleo – I recommend soaking them in water overnight then drying them out on a sheet pan in the sunlight. (Or over a heater / radiator if it's winter time.) If you have a bit of time over the weekend, it's best to prepare your nuts this way so you can use them whenever you want. Even beans and legumes can be prepared for immediate use, but those must be kept in the fridge or else they will keep on sprouting!

Prep time: 5 min. + 6-12 hours to soak and dehydrate the almonds if you're Paleo
Cook time: 20 min.
Storage time: Up to 5 days in the fridge or 3 months in the freezer
Suitable diets: Gluten-Free, Vegan, Vegetarian, Paleo
Servings: 3

Calories*: 461 kcal
Protein*: 13.5 g
Carbs*: 24.9 g
Fat*: 38 g (3.2 grams of which saturates)
*Per portion

Ingredients:
- 1 pound of string beans (thin or "French style" green beans)
- ½ medium-sized yellow onion
- 1 fresh lemon
- 1 ½ cup almonds
- 1 tablespoon Bragg's Amino Acids (or the same amount of soy sauce, or 3 pinches of salt)
- 3 tablespoons avocado oil or sunflower oil

Instructions:

- After soaking the almonds overnight and letting them dehydrate / dry out, place them in a frying pan *without oil* on medium-low heat. Let toast for 5-8 minutes, stirring occasionally. Watch them carefully so they don't burn.
- Meanwhile, trim the green beans and slice at a steep diagonal, into bite-sized pieces. Chop the onion.
- Take a medium-sized frying pan, put in the oil and onion and beans. Sautée for 10 minutes, until the beans are *al dente* and the onion is translucent. Add the almonds, juice from the lemon (or ¼ cup lemon juice from a bottle), Bragg's Amino Acids, and stir well, cooking for another 2 minutes.
- Serve warm as a side dish, adding salt and pepper to taste.

Mashed Cauliflower with Garlic

You might be surprised that this recipe serves 9, when most other recipes I've included in this book serve 2-4 as a rule. The reason is simple: Everyone will LOVE this healthy new spin on mashed potatoes! If your family doesn't go back for second helpings/servings, then you can easily freeze the rest for up to two months.

Prep time: 10 min.
Cook time: 20 min.
Storage time: Up to 3 days in the fridge or 3 months in the freezer
Suitable diets: Gluten-Free, Vegan, Vegetarian, Paleo
Servings: 9 (that's not a typo!)

Calories*: 134 kcal
Protein*: 5.5 g
Carbs*: 14.5 g
Fat*: 7.6 g (5.7 grams of which saturates)
*Per portion

Ingredients:
- 3 heads cauliflower
- 6 tablespoon(s) vegan butter* (or olive oil)
- 4.5-6 cloves garlic* (minced)
- ~0.75 teaspoon(s) sea salt (to taste)
- 1.5 pinch black pepper
- 0.38 - 0.75 cup unsweetened plain almond milk (to help with pureeing)
- Fresh parsley and chives to serve (optional)

Instructions:
Cut the cauliflower into small, bite-sized pieces and place into a large pot. Put 2 inches of water at the bottom, to steam. Let steam for 15-20 minutes or until *al dente.*

While that is steaming, press the garlic and margarine into a small frying pan, and sautée over medium-low heat for 2-3 minutes or until mixture has just slightly turned brown (be careful not to burn).

Put approximately half the cauliflower mixture into a food processor or blender or use a stick blender and mix until puréed smooth. Then, add half the garlic butter, the salt, and the pepper. Continue mixing well.

Feel free to add some extra almond milk to help the cauliflower purée get more watery or creamy, and less thick. You could add a couple pinches of nutritional yeast to add some cheesy flavor if you'd like.

Transfer the mixture to a large bowl or serving platter. Keep it warm in the oven on low heat. Repeat the blending and seasoning of the cauliflower mixture until you've used up all your ingredients.

To serve, sprinkle some freshly chopped chives or parsley on top. Add freshly ground pepper to taste.

Spicy Cauliflower Burgers

If you're on a Paleo diet, these make wonderful bases to put Ratatouille atop, or simply enjoy on their own. Once you get a bit creative with vegetables, it's so much easier to think outside the (bread)box and leave those buns behind!

Prep time: 20 min.
Cook time: 10 min.
Storage time: Up to 2 days in the fridge or 1 month in the freezer
Suitable diets: Gluten-Free, Vegan, Vegetarian, Paleo
Servings: 5

Calories*: 83 kcal (that's not a typo!)
Protein*: 4.5 g
Carbs*: 17.7 g
Fat*: 0.4 g (0.1 gram of which saturates)
*Per portion

Ingredients:
8 cups cauliflower (this is about 1 large head)
1 tablespoon(s) baking powder
2 teaspoon(s) of dried oregano
½ teaspoon(s) of garlic powder
⅔ cup flour (spelt, white, oat, almond, whichever you'd like to use)
2 dashes of Himalayan finely ground salt
¼ cup + 2 tablespoon(s) water

Instructions:
Chop the cauliflower into bite-size pieces. Put into a pot with an inch or two of water at the bottom, and into a steamer basket if you have one. Steam the cauliflower until it is soft enough that you can poke it with a fork.

Drain the water from the pot. Once the cauliflower has cooled, place it on to a clean towel or cheesecloth. Place that over a bowl, or over the sink. Press it gently so as much water comes out of it as possible.

Place the cauliflower in a large bowl. Whisk together all the other ingredients in a separate bowl, then add those whisked-together ingredients to the cauliflower. Mash all of it very well with a spoon.

Shape into patties with your hands. I usually make a medium-sized 'snow ball' shape, and then flatten it. To cook, fry the patties in 2-3 tablespoons of veggie oil on medium heat for about 5 minutes on each side. Or, bake in the oven on 400°F / gas mark 6 for 10-12 minutes. Flip, and bake another 10 minutes or until lightly brown and crispy.

Vietnamese Summer Rolls

These are a great, light, veggie-packed alternative to deep fat fried spring rolls. If you cannot find rice paper sheets for the outside of the roll, feel free to use Romaine lettuce leaves or another creative solution to wrap up the delicious vegetable ingredients.

Prep time: 20 min.
Cook time: 10 min.
Storage time: Up to 2 days in the fridge or 1 month in the freezer
Suitable diets: Gluten-Free, Vegan, Vegetarian, Paleo
Servings: About 20

Calories*: 59 kcal
Protein*: 0.9 g
Carbs*: 11.6 g
Fat*: 1.3 g (0.2 gram of which saturates)
*Per portion

Ingredients:
- 2 ounce pack of rice papers
- dipping sauce of your choice to serve (I usually mix equal parts of smooth peanut butter with water, and a teaspoon of lime juice and a tablespoon of fresh cilantro)
- 3 ½ ounces rice vermicelli
- 1 carrot
- 1 cucumber
- ½ mango (or half of a can of mango)*
- ⅔ cup cherry tomatoes
- 1/3 cup roasted peanuts
- 1 handful of fresh mint leaves
- 1 handful of Thai basil or cilantro
- 1 fresh lime, or bottled lime juice to sprinkle atop to serve
  *If you're following a properly combined food diet, substitute the mango

Instructions:

Pour some boiling water over the rice vermicelli and leave it for a few minutes until it's rehydrated but not too soggy. (This takes about 10 minutes.) This is a great time to prepare your vegetables and other ingredients.

Cut the carrot into very thin slices or 'batons', long and thin sticks. Cut the cucumber and mango the same way. Halve the cherry tomatoes and crush the roasted peanuts. Chop the fresh mint leaves and basil into long strips – remember, the longer the veggie mixture, the less likely it is to fall out of the summer roll when you bit into it!

To make the summer roles, drain the vermicelli and then pour your dressing over the noodles and let them soak further (marinate) for about 15 minutes.

Prepare a bowl of cold water large enough for you to submerge a rice paper into. Set it aside with a damp, clean cloth.

Take rice paper and submerge it in the bowl of cold water, then place it on top of the damp cloth for 10-15 seconds. You want it to be moist, but not so wet that it'll tear when handling it.

Place the marinated noodles to one side of the rice paper, a bit off-center. Add a few slices of the carrot, cucumber, mango, tomatoes, peanuts and herbs. Tuck in the shorter edges and roll.

<u>Note for beginners:</u> Be careful to not add too much mixture into each roll. "Less is more" so that they stay tightly rolled together and don't fall apart.

Roll the rest of the rice papers until you've used up all your ingredients. The exact number of summer rolls depends on the size of cucumber, carrot and other ingredients you use, and how full you fill the rolls, too. Serve with your sauce (or a canned sauce) and fresh lime juice sprinkled atop.

[4.6] Beans, Peas, Seeds & More

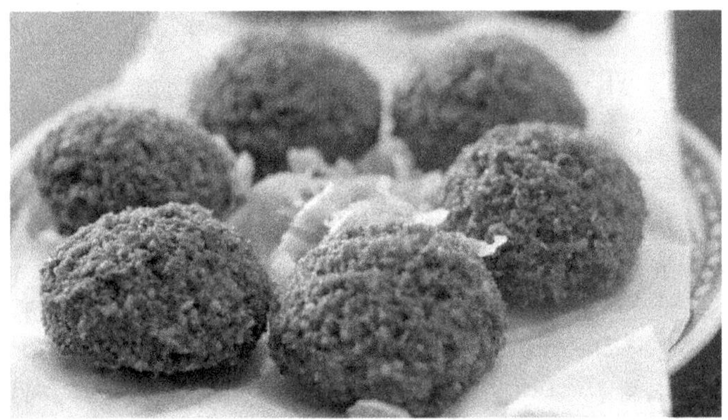

Chickpea-Free Falafel with Coriander

Prep time: 20 min.
Soak time: 30 min.
Dehydrate time: overnight or 8 hours
Storage: 2 days in the fridge
Serves: 4

Calories*: 301 kcal
Protein*: 9.2 g
Carbs*: 8 g
Fat*: 26.1 g (3.7 grams of which saturates)
*Per portion

Ingredients:
- ½ cup sunflower seeds
- 1/3 cup pumpkin seeds
- 2 tablespoons coriander leaves
- ½ teaspoon ground coriander

- ½ teaspoon ground cumin
- 6 sun-dried tomatoes (not halves, as they usually come in jars)
- 1 garlic clove
- 1 shallot
- ½ cup green or black olives (without the pits)
- 2 pinches of smoked, powdered paprika
- 2 pinches of finely ground Himalaya salt
- 1 handful of salad leaves to serve

TAHINI CREAM
- 3 tablespoons tahini (sesame paste)
- 2 teaspoons xylitol
- 2 tablespoons lemon juice
- pinch of Himalaya salt

Instructions:

Place all the falafel ingredients in a food processor and process until completely mixed. Shape the falafel mixture with your hands into walnut-sized balls and place directly on a mesh dehydrator sheet or a baking sheet.

Put into the dehydrator set to 115°F, or place in the oven at the lowest temperature possible, 115°F -- if your oven is too hot, then leave the door ajar (open) slightly overnight or for 8 hours. They should be firm to the touch.

To make the tahini cream, place all the ingredients in a blender with 2 tablespoons of lukewarm water and blend until smooth and creamy. To serve, place the salad leaves on a platter, top with the falafel and drizzle over the cream.

Hearty Italian Bean & Barley Stew

Prep time: 5 min.
Cook time: 20-28 min.
Storage time: Up to 7 days in the fridge or 6 months in the freezer
Suitable diets: Gluten-Free, Vegan, Vegetarian, Paleo, Low-Sugar
Servings: 4 adult-size portions

Calories*: 196 kcal
Protein*: 7.6 g
Carbs*: 25.5 g
Fat*: 7.8 g (2.3 grams of which saturates, depending on which soup stock you use)
*Per portion

Ingredients:

- 2 tablespoons extra virgin olive oil
- 1 garlic clove
- 2 carrots
- 2 celery
- 1 large leek
- 1 quart vegetable stock
- 1 tablespoon of tomato purée
- 3 tablespoons pearl barley (**<u>remember to soak the barley</u>** for 6 hours if you're Paleo!)
- 1 can of beans (white, butter, kidney, or pinto)
- 2 cups of leafy greens
- bread to serve (optional)

Instructions:

Heat 2 tablespoons of olive oil in a large pan on medium heat. Chop the garlic, carrots, celery and leeks. Add to the pan and cook until they soften.

Add the soup stock or boullión, tomato purée and barley. Let cook for a minute or two, until it's all heated up again, then turn onto low heat and let simmer for 15-20 minutes. The barley should just turn tender. (You can poke it with a fork or press with the back of a spoon.)

Add the beans and greens and simmer for 5 more minutes. Serve with crusty bread if you'd like, or the gluten-free, raw bread recipe in this book. Salt and pepper to taste.

Pea Soup

Prep time: 5 min.
Cook time: 15 min.
Storage time: Up to 7 days in the fridge or 6 months in the freezer
Suitable diets: Gluten-Free, Vegan, Vegetarian, Paleo, Low-Sugar
Servings: 4 adult-size portions

Calories*: 183 kcal
Protein*: 5.6 g
Carbs*: 29.8 g
Fat*: 4.5 g (0.9 grams of which saturates, depending on which soup stock you use)
*Per portion

Ingredients:
- 1 onion
- 3 cloves garlic
- 1 large potato or 2 smaller ones
- 2 cups of peas, fresh or frozen
- 3 quarts of vegetable broth or water with some salt
- 1 tbsp vegetable oil
- Salt, pepper to taste
- fresh herbs to taste: parsley, lovage
- 1 tbsp lemon juice
- fresh thyme (just a teaspoon or a dash)
- chopped peanuts (about a handful)

Instructions:
Finely chop the onion and garlic cloves. Then, dice the potato. (I leave the skins on, because most of the nutritional content in them.) In a large pot, heat one tablespoon of veggie oil or sunflower oil. Add onion and garlic, sautéeing until translucent, stirring occasionally. Add diced potatoes and peas (you can add them

straight from the freezer, that's OK), pour in the vegetable stock and season with Himalaya salt, freshly ground pepper and finely chopped fresh herbs to taste.

Let it simmer on low heat for about 15 minutes, until the potatoes and peas are tender enough you can pierce through them with a fork. Then, remove from heat, add a tablespoon of lemon juice and blend until smooth in a blender (or with a stick blender).

To serve, pour in a bit of soy cream and stir lightly. This gives it a wonderful color contrast.

[4.7] Legumes (Potatoes & Nuts)

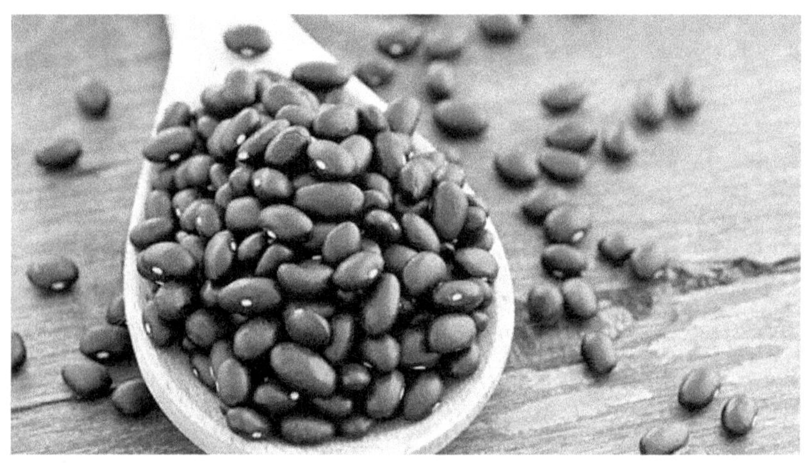

Sweet Potato Chili with Quinoa

Prep time: 15 min.
Cook time: 30 min.
Storage time: Up to 6 days in the fridge
Suitable diets: Vegan, Vegetarian
Servings: 4

Calories*: 388 kcal
Protein*: 12.1 g
Carbs*: 65.3 g
Fat*: 5.8 g (0.7 grams of which saturates)

Ingredients:
- onion 1 large, finely chopped
- garlic 2 cloves, crushed
- olive oil

- mild chilli powder 1 tablespoon(s)
- ground cumin 1 teaspoon(s)
- 3 medium sweet potatoes, peeled and cubed
- 1 cup quinoa, and drained
- 1 can of chopped tomatoes
- 2 quarts of vegetable stock
- 1 can of black beans, rinsed and drained
- coriander a small bunch, to serve
- soured cream or yogurt to serve (optional)

Instructions:

Take a large pot. Dice the onion. Cook the onion and garlic in 1 tablespoon(s) olive oil until soft. Add the chilli powder and cumin, cook for a minute then add the sweet potato, quinoa, tomatoes and stock. Let simmer for about 10 minutes, then put in the beans. Half cover the pot with a lid, letting it simmer for maybe 20 to 30 more minutes. The squash and quinoa should be soft enough to poke through with a fork. The liquid should also be noticeably thicker. Sprinkle over the coriander you've chopped up and serve in bowls with a dollop of soured cream or yogurt if you like.

Spicy Sweet Potato Enchiladas

Prep time: 10 min.
Cook time: 20 min.
Storage time: Up to 6 days in the fridge
Suitable diets: Vegan, Vegetarian
Servings: 6

Calories*: 495 kcal
Protein*: 13.9 g
Carbs*: 60.7 g
Fat*: 19.4 g (7.2 grams of which saturates)

I recommend making more of the sauce (triple the batch) and freezing it for future use.

Ingredients:

- 1 large sweet potatoes
- 1 red or yellow onion 1
- 1 red bell pepper
- 1 green bell pepper
- 1 teaspoons cumin seeds
- 1 teaspoon dried chilli flakes
- 3 tablespoons olive oil
- 1 small bunch of cilantro / coriander
- 4 large tortillas
- 1 ½ cups grated vegan cheese
- sour cream to serve
- salad to serve

ENCHILADA SAUCE
1 can chopped tomatoes
1 teaspoon smoked paprika

1 teaspoon garlic salt (or use half Himalaya salt, half garlic powder)

1 teaspoon dried oregano

1 teaspoon sugar

Heat the oven to 200°C / 400°F /gas mark 6. Chop all of the fresh ingredients, leaving the skins on the potatoes. Finely chop the herbs.

Put the potatoes, onion, bell peppers / capsicum and spices on a non-stick baking tray or a baking sheet lined with wax parchment paper. Add the oil and lots of salt and pepper, and toss well. Cook for half an hour or until the potato is tender enough to pierce with a fork (but not mushy).

Meanwhile, blend the sauce ingredients together in a blender. Take the veg out of the oven and leave to cool a little. Stir through ½ the coriander.

Lay out the tortillas flat and spread out the veggie mixture evenly between them. Roll up the tortillas; you may want to look up a video on the internet for this, as it helps to watch. Place the tortillas cutside down into an oiled baking dish.

Spoon over the sauce and sprinkle over the cheese, using the nut cheese recipe that we have in this chapter if you'd like. Put them in the oven and bake for about 20 minutes or until bubbling and golden. Serve with vegan sour cream, the other half of the chopped coriander and a fresh side salad.

Raw Nut Cheese

You can use almonds instead of cashews, or a mixture of the two. Macadamia nuts work well, but don't have much of the same flavor as the other two. Feel free to experiment with adding shallots (spring onions), chives, or other herbs. This cheese substitute is also a great probiotic food to re-balance the bowel flora in the gut.

<u>Don't forget to soak the cashews overnight!</u>

Prep time: 10 min. + 12 hours soak time + 12 hours set / rise time

Cook time: 0 min.

Storage time: Up to 7 days in the fridge

Suitable diets: Vegan, Vegetarian, Raw, Paleo, Properly Combined

Servings: 3

Calories*: 890 kcal

Protein*: 36 g

Carbs*: 59.7 g

Fat*: 65 g (13 grams of which saturates)

Ingredients:

- 3 ⅔ cups raw cashews
- 1 teaspoon of probiotic powder
- 2 tablespoons onion powder
- 1 tablespoon garlic powder
- 4-5 tablespoons nutritional yeast
- salt and pepper to taste

Instructions:

Drain the water from the overnight soaked cashews. Put them in a blender with the probiotic powder, blending until smooth.

Transfer the mixture into a bowl and cover with plastic wrap or beeswax wrap, being careful to leave a couple tiny spaces open for air to get in. Leave the bowl at room temperature for 8-12 hours, or until the cheese has risen in size and taken on an airated quality.

111

Season to taste with the onion powder, garlic powder, nutritional yeast, salt, and pepper. It's wonderful on crackers, or sprinkled / grated atop any pasta dish to make a vegan, perfectly combined meal.

[4.8] Cereals & Grains

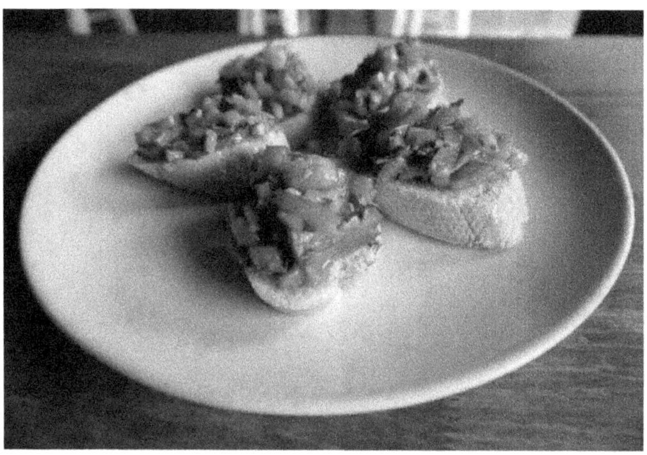

Italian Tomatoes on Toast ("Bruschetta")

I was originally using sourdough for this quick and easy recipe, because the flavor accentuates the tomatoes and vinegar very well. Feel free to use the gluten-free bread in the recipe above, or any style you like that has flavor and 'character' as we say in Italy!

This is a great recipe for breakfast because it's so quick and easy to prepare. It's both light and filling at the same time, giving you enough energy for your morning but not bogging down your stomach with lots to digest.

Prep time: 5 min.

Cook time: 5 min.

Storage time: none – it gets soggy after about an hour, so consume immediately

Suitable diets: Vegan, Vegetarian

Servings: 2

Calories*: 212 kcal (depending largely on the type of bread you choose to use)
Protein*: 6.4 g
Carbs*: 40.4 g
Fat*: 2.8 g (0.5 grams of which saturates)
*Per serving

Ingredients:

- 2 large, ripe tomatoes
- 1 teaspoon red wine vinegar / sherry vinegar OR 1 tablespoon red wine
- 4 thin slices of sourdough bread (or the gluten-free, paleo recipe I've written earlier)
- ½ garlic clove
- 1 teaspoon extra virgin olive oil
- Himalayan salt and ground black pepper to taste

Money Saving Tip: If you have any red wine left over, save it in a jar or small bowl. If left uncovered, it will oxidize – essentially turning into the same taste as vinegar! White wine is better for some recipes, but red will taste very similar, too.

Instructions:

Begin toasting the bread on a hot griddle, or slightly warm the paleo bread you've made from the recipe above it if you're following a raw diet.

Wash and chop the tomatoes. I usually remove the inner part with the seeds, keeping them for soup or muffins. (Leftover or 'discarded' bits of food actually keep quite well in the freezer!)

Mix the tomatoes with the vinegar, salt and pepper.

Press the garlic, crushing it into a fine pulp. Spread very thinly on the toast. Top the toast with the tomatoes and add a bit of olive oil on top of each. Consume immediately. (I sometimes add a sprinkle of chopped basil or parsley on top as well, for extra Vitamin C and trace minerals. The extra color also looks quite nice.)

Gluten-Free, Raw Bread with Caraway Onion

Remember to soak the seeds and walnuts overnight, or for at least 6 hours. This is not only good for a Paleo diet, but makes them more supple for grinding and shaping into falafel.

Prep time: 15 min.
Soak time: 4-6 hours
Storage: 2 weeks in an airtight container
Serves: 4

Suitable diets: Paleo, Vegan, Vegetarian, Gluten-Free, Raw

Ingredients:
- 4 ½ ounces sunflower seeds
- 3 ounces walnuts
- 3 celery stalks
- 2 ounces raisins (soak these for at least 2 hours)
- 1 red onion
- 2 teaspoons caraway seeds
- 2 tablespoons ground coriander
- 2 pinches Himalayan salt
- 3 ounces ground flaxseeds
- 4 ounces extra virgin olive oil
- 4 tablespoons lemon juice

Instructions:
Soak the seeds and nuts overnight or for 4-6 hours. Drain the water. Dice the onion, celery and chop the seeds. Add all into a blender or food processor and mix very well for 2-5 minutes or until well blended. Add the rest of the ingredients.

Pat out flat on a baking tray lined with wax paper, or put into a dehydrator. Bake / dehydrate for 6 hours (baking at 115°F or the lowest setting with door ajar).

Flaxseed Crackers with Sundried Tomatoes

In lieu of an "Italian herb" spice mix, you can make it yourself with dried basil, parsley, oregano, and garlic.

Prep time: 5 min.
Dehydration time: 25 hours
Soak time: 2-4 hours
Suitable diets: Raw, Gluten-Free, Vegan, Vegetarian, Paleo

Calories*: 169 kcal
Protein*: 6.4 g
Carbs*: 10.9 g
Fat*: 11.6 g (1.1 grams of which saturates)
*Per serving

Ingredients:
- 10 ½ ounces whole flaxseeds
- 1 ¼ pints water
- 8 ½ ounces sunflower seeds
- 1 ½ ounces fresh basil
- 10 sun-dried tomatoes (or 20 halves)
- 1 red pepper (the hot, spicy kind)
- 1 tablespoon of chia seeds
- 2 tablespoons of mixed Italian herbs
- 1 tablespoon of garlic powder
- 2 pinches of Himalayan salt

Instructions:
Stir the flaxseed with water and leave to soak for 2-4 hours.

Put all the ingredients, except the soaking flax seeds, in a food processor with an S blade and process until the mixture resembles a thick soup. Add the flax and process to combine.

Divide the mixture into 2 portions and spread each over a Teflex sheet. Use a spatula to bring the mixture as close as you can to the edges of the sheet without it separating. Dehydrate at 48°C for 10 hours.

Place a mesh tray over 1 cracker and, holding the tray and the Teflex sheet together at each end, quickly invert the stack, then peel off the Teflex sheet. Repeat with the other racker. Dehydrate on the trays at 48!C for 15 hours.

Chop up the large planks of cracker into equally sized squares and store them in an airtight container.

[4.9] Desserts & Sweets

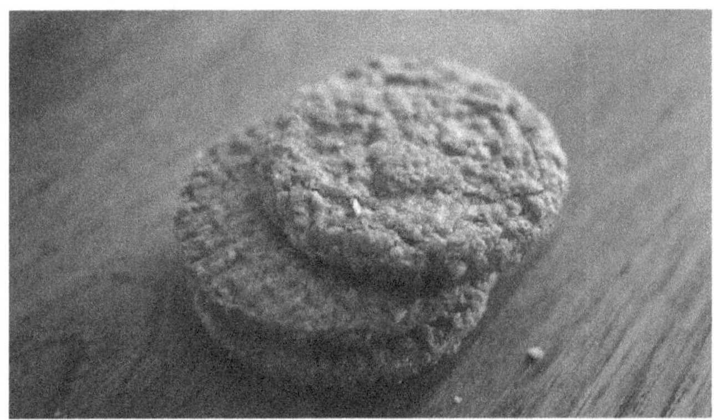

It's important to note that the ingredients, brand names and foods listed here are designed for a US audience. What we call baking soda is called bicarbonate of soda in the UK, for example. I've done my best to add asterisks and small notes where these differences pop up.

Anti-Inflammatory Apple Cinnamon Cookies

Prep time: 10 min.
Dehydration time: 20 hours
Suitable diets: Raw, Vegan, Vegetarian, Gluten-Free, Low-Sugar
Servings: About 12

Ingredients:
- 2 medium-sized apples

- 2 ½ ounces pitted dates
- 6 ½ ground almonds or almond meal (the pulp left over after making almond milk)
- 4 ½ ounces cashew nuts
- 3 tablespoons coconut palm sugar
- 3 tablespoons ground cinnamon
- 1 pinch of finely ground Himalayan salt

Instructions:

Put the apples and dates in a food processor and blend to a paste. You may have to chop the apples into large chunks first to fit them inside. Add the remaining ingredients and process to a grainy dough.

Transfer the mixture to a Teflex sheet, cover with another sheet and press down on the top sheet to smooth out the dough. When it is about ¼ inch thick, peel off the top sheet. Stamp out biscuits using cookie cutters, leaving the offcuts intact.

Dehydrate at 48°C for 10 hours, turn over onto a mesh tray and dehydrate for 8-10 hours. Discard the offcuts.

Anti-Inflammatory Ginger Tonic

Ginger, just like cinnamon, is well-known for its anti-inflammatory properties. Civilizations around the world have been using it for centuries to ease gout, arthritis and other inflammatory conditions.

This tonic or "alcohol-free ginger beer" is a quick one to make, needing only 24 hours to set. You'll need some dry yeast, because it acts as a fermenting agent. Yeast – the good kind – has an antimicrobial effect in the gut. Rather than relying on cow-milk yogurts for 'good bacteria' for the gut – or even worse, buying expensive probiotic supplements – simply get in the habit of drinking more fermented, homemade drinks.

Make sure you use very clean glass bottles to store the tonic. And it's best stored cold in the refrigerator, because yeast will continue to rise and grow in warm temperatures or even at room temperature. Oh, and active dried yeast is completely paleo, too!

Prep time: 5 min.
Cook time: 5 min.
Brew time: 1 day
Storage time: 2-3 weeks in the fridge
Suitable diets: Vegan, Vegetarian, Paleo, Low-Sugar
Servings: 3

Nutritional information: I haven't included any, because this recipe largely relies upon the kind of sweetener you choose to use. I often use honey, but if you're a strict vegan then you can substitute white granulated sugar or coconut blossom nectar / syrup in lieu of honey. Maple syrup, agave and stevia also work, but the yeast needs more time to grow with those substances that have less sugar although they taste just as sweet.

Ingredients:
- 1 quart of boiling water
- ½ cup honey (or a heaping ½ cup of white sugar)
- 1 fresh lemon (try to buy organic)
- 1 chunk of ginger roughly the size of your thumb (or more, if you like it spicier)
- 1 teaspoon dried yeast

Instructions:
Bring the water to a boil.

Have you heard of the saying "a watched pot never boils"? By now you should know that the art of cooking involves multi-tasking and timing. So while you're waiting for the water to boil, squeeze the juice from your lemon. Keep the peel.

Peel the skin off the ginger with a teaspoon – this leaves a lot more 'flesh' on the ginger root than if you would use a knife. Slice it into thin pieces.

Remove the boiling water from heat as soon as it's reached a boil. Let it cool so that you can touch the outside of the pan. (Did you know? If yeast is put into boiling water, it dies.) After it's cooled, add the yeast, honey / sugar, ginger slices, juice from the entire lemon, and the lemon peel. Cover the mixture with a muslin cloth or plastic wrap / cling film. (I use beeswax wraps at home and love them! They're reusable and last a very long time if you touch them up with a bit of way every few months.)

Leave covered at room temperature for 24 hours. Skim off any scum that has risen to the top. Strain the liquid through a sieve to remove any lemon pulp, ginger chunks, and the lemon peel. Pour into glass bottles or jars, leaving a little room at the top. Keep well chilled in your fridge and serve these over ice with a slice of fresh lemon on the side. Tip for adults: Dark spiced rum goes very well with this drink if you'd prefer an adult version in the evening!

Chocolate Chunk & Apricot Cookie Bars

Prep time: 20 min.
Cook time: 0 min.
Storage time: Up to 5 days in the fridge
Suitable diets: Raw, Vegan, Vegetarian
Servings: 12 bars

Calories*: 196 kcal
Protein*: 4.9 g
Carbs*: 11.2 g
Fat*: 15.3 g (3 grams of which saturates)
Per bar, recipe makes 12 bars

Ingredients:

- 1 ¼ cup pecans
- 2 tablespoons whole flaxseeds
- ¾ heaping cup cashew nuts
- pinch of cinnamon
- 2 tablespoons raw cacao powder
- pinch of sea salt
- 1 scant cup dried, ready-to-eat apricots
- 4 tablespoons raw cacao nibs

Instructions:

Place the pecans and flaxseeds that you've already soaked and drained into a blender, and blend until finely chopped. Repeat with the cashew nuts, allowing some of the nuts to remain coarsely chopped for texture. Place in a bowl. Add the cinnamon, cacao powder and salt.

Place the apricots in a food processor and process to form a thick purée, then add to the nut mixture to form a dough. Stir in the cacao nibs.

Spread the mixture into a rectangle about ½ inch thick on a non-stick sheet placed on a baking or dehydrator tray. Mark into bars and put into a dehydrator set at 115°F or place in an oven at 115°F or on its lowest setting with the door ajar. Let dehydrate for 6 hours. Flip them over and dry them for another 2-4 hours. The mixture should still be chewy. Alternatively, press the mixture into a shallow tin lined with cling film / saran wrap, then mark into bars. Freeze until firm for about 3-4 hours, then move to the fridge for 1 hour before eating.

Blueberry Chocolate Torta

Prep time: 30 min. + 2-3 hours chilling time
Soaking time: 15 min.
Storage: 3-4 days in the fridge or 1 month in the freezer
Servings: 10

Calories: 280 kcal
Protein: 3.4 g
Carbohydrates: 12.7 g
Fat: 24.7 g (9.9 g of which saturates)
*Per portion

Ingredients

- 1 ½ cup pecans
- 1 fresh lemon
- ½ cup pitted dates
- 3 tablespoons melted coconut butter
- ½ cup cashew nuts
- 1/3 heaping cup of raw cacao powder
- 4 ounces cacao butter
- 1 tablespoons xylitol or stevia (or other powdered sweetener)
- 2 cups of blueberries (fresh is better)

Instructions:

Place the pecans in a blender and blend until finely chopped. Place in a bowl with the lemon zest. Place the dates in the blender with the coconut butter and blend to form a purée. Stir into the pecans to form a dough. Press into an 8 inch springform cake pan and chill.

Place the cashew nuts, cacao powder, cacao butter, xylitol, lemon juice and blueberries in a food processor and process until smooth. Fold in the strawberries.

Spread over the crust and chill for 2-3 hours until set.

Lemon Pistachio Cookies

This recipe is one of my kids' favorites to bake. Children love the sensory play of squeezing out fresh juice from the lemon and forming little balls from the dough by rolling it in between the palms of their hands.

Prep time: 30 min.
Bake time: 12 min.
Storage time: Up to 10 days in an airtight container or 6 months in the freezer
Suitable diets: Vegan, Vegetarian
Servings: 16 cookies

Calories*: 201 kcal
Protein*: 3.2 g
Carbs*: 28.1 g
Fat*: 8.8 g (0.9 grams of which saturates)
*Per portion

Ingredients:
- 3 cups whole-wheat pastry flour or wholemeal bread flour
- ½ teaspoon baking soda (or "bicarbonate of soda")
- ½ teaspoon ground cinnamon
- ½ teaspoon finely ground Himalaya salt

- 1 fresh lemon, using juice from half of it, and half or two-thirds of the lemon's zest*
- ⅔ cup sunflower oil
- ⅔ cup maple syrup
- ½ teaspoon almond extract
- 1 cup shelled and chopped pistachios
- baking sheet and wax baking paper or parchment paper

Zest of a fruit is a fancy name for its peel that's been finely grated. It has a bitter taste, so add less if it's your first time baking with any citrus fruit zest. Also, because pesticides are often in the peels and outsides of produce, try to buy an organic lemon for this recipe.

Instructions:

Preheat the oven to 375°F while you chop the pistachios and place them into a frying pan. Toast the pistachios without oil or butter, simply on medium heat in the pan or skillet until they've taken on a golden brown color on the edges. (Careful not to burn them! Stir often.)

In a large bowl, combine the dry ingredients and stir until they are well mixed, smooth and even.

In a separate bowl, combine the wet ingredients and whisk well until smooth. Add the wet ingredients to the dry bit by bit, making sure to pause and stir well before adding some more. Doing this ensures you won't have lumps in your cookie dough.

Add the toasted pistachios last, folding them in. "Folding" is a fancy term saying you shouldn't stir too much. Add some pistachios, cover that with some more dough, add more pistachios, and repeat until the nuts are evenly "folded in" or spread throughout the dough mixture.

Using your hands, form the dough into little balls that are approximately one inch in diameter (through the middle). Set on the baking sheet and press down with your thumb to flatten them, making sure that they are roughly the same height throughout the entire cookie (or else they might burn on the thin edges!). Bake for 10-12 minutes, or until they have a light golden brown color on the bottom. Cool them on the baking sheet for a couple minutes, then transfer them to a wire cooling rack to cool completely. The reason

I don't let baked goods cool in their pans or sheets is because the hot metal continues to cook the cake or cookie whilst it's cooling, thereby drying it out a bit too much.

[4.10] Quick Snacks & Smoothies

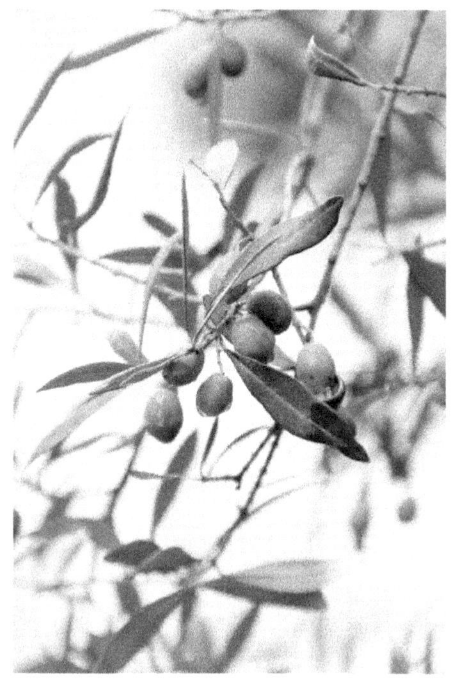

If you're serious about eating a healthy, plant-based diet, then you'll likely invest in a dehydrator at some point. I've gotten into the habit of preparing lots of fruits for overnight dehydration:

Pineapple can be used straight out of the can, and apples with a sprinkle of cinnamon on top make especially delicious substitutes for salty, fat-laden chips.

Also don't forget your veggie staples! Carrots, sweet potato, and parsnips make delightful crunchy chips when dehydrated – but you'll want to boil them first to bring out their sweet flavor.

Hummus with Olives & Pine Nuts

Prep time: 30 min.
Bake time: 12 min.
Storage time: Up to 10 days in an airtight container or 6 months in the freezer
Suitable diets: Vegan, Vegetarian
Servings: 16 cookies
Calories*: 392 kcal
Protein*: 11.4 g
Carbs*: 23.5 g
Fat*: 26.2 g (3.3 grams of which saturates)
*Per portion

Ingredients:

- 1 can of large chickpeas, drained (1 tablespoon(s) of the liquid reserved)
- 4 tablespoons tahini
- 3 garlic cloves
- 4 tablespoons extra-virgin olive oil (and some more to sprinkle on top for garnish)
- 1-2 tablespoons fresh lemon juice
- 1½ tablespoon(s) of raisins
- 1½ tablespoon(s) of pine nuts
- ½ teaspoon(s) of cumin seeds

- 12-15 pitted kalamata olives
- 1 tablespoon of chopped flat-leaf parsley
- pittas or flatbreads to serve

Instructions:

Put the chickpeas / garbanzo beans and tahini in a food processor. (I remove the shells from the chickpeas, but it's tedious. You can leave them on for a slightly more bitter taste.) Sautée the pressed garlic and 2 tablespoon(s) of the oil in a small skillet over medium heat for about 2 minutes.

Put the garlic and oil into a food processor. Add 1 tablespoon(s) of the lemon juice and reserved chickpea liquid, plus ¼ teaspoon(s) sea salt and some pepper. Blend until really smooth, then taste and add more salt, pepper, olive oil and lemon juice if needed.

Put the rest of the oil and garlic into the frying pan you've just used. Sautée on low heat until the garlic just starts sizzling, then add the raisins, pine nuts and cumin. Cook it all for about 5 minutes, until the raisins are softening and pine nuts browning.

Warm the hummus in a small pan, then spread it over a plate or put into a bowl, then sprinkle over the raisins and nuts. Eat with bread.

Chia Coconut Granola-Free Bars

Prep time: 30 minutes, plus 2 hours chilling time
Soaking time: 10 min.
Storage: 1 week in the fridge or 1 month in the freezer
Servings: 18 bars

Calories: 209 kcal
Protein: 3.6 g
Carbs: 12.8 g
Fat: 16.1 g (or which saturates 7.8 g)

Ingredients:
- 1 ¼ heaping cup of almonds
- 2 heaping tablespoons of chia seeds
- 2 cups dried mango
- 1 orange
- 2 tablespoons xylitol or stevia powdered sweetener
- 4 tablespoons melted coconut butter
- pinch of Himalaya salt
- 3 tablespoons lucuma powder
- 1/3 cup ground flaxseeds
- 1 1/3 cups desiccated / flaked coconut

Instructions:

Place the almonds in a blender and blend to a fine flour. Repeat with the chia seeds.

Place half the mango in a blender with the chia powder, orange juice, xylitol, melted coconut butter and salt. Blend to form a thick purée. Finely chop the remaining mango.

Put the lucuma powder, ground almonds (or almond meal), mango pieces, ground flaxseeds, and three-quarters of the coconut into a large-sized bowl. Pour in the contents you've just blended, and stir until everything is well mixed together.

Sprinkle a scant handful of the remaining coconut onto a sheet of waxed baking parchment, that is on a baking tray. 12 x 8 inches should work just fine.

Press the mixture onto the baking tray and flatten. Sprinkle all that's left of the coconut flakes on top, and press everything down firmly. Chill for 2 hours or until firm, then cut into bars.

Chocolate Superfood Protein Balls

Prep time: 20 min.
Soaking time: 10 min.
Storage: 3-4 days in the fridge
Servings: 16 balls

Calories: 135 kcal
Protein: 2.5 g
Carbs: 11.8 g
Fat: 8.7 g (3.1 g of which saturates)

Ingredients:
- 1 ¼ cups pecans
- 1 tablespoon lucuma powder
- 1 tablespoon maca powder
- 4 tablespoons raw cacao powder
- 2 tablespoons xylitol
- 1 tablespoon flower pollen granules
- ½ cup goji berries
- 10 pitted dates
- 3 tablespoons coconut butter
- desiccated / flaked coconut for rolling the ball in

Instructions:

Place the pecans, lucuma powder, maca powder, cacao powder and xylitol in a blender or food processor and process to form a fine powder. Place in a bowl with the flower pollen.

Place the dried fruit and coconut butter in the blender or food processor and process to form a sticky paste - still keeping some texture. Knead into the dry ingredients to form a stiff dough.

Form into balls then roll in the desiccated coconut.

Chocolate Berry Smoothie

You don't have to feel guilty indulging in this chocolate smoothie because it's packed with antioxidants from the berries and chocolate. I've added some vegan pea protein powder for the extra health kick. And did you know? Frozen berries have just as much – if not more – vitamin content than their fresh siblings. Because they're frozen and stored in air-tight containers, the air and sunshine and heat, which are all factors that destroy Vitamin C easily, cannot damage any vitamins.

Prep time: 3 minutes
Cook time: under one minute
Storage time: Up to 4 days in the fridge or 3 months in the freezer
Suitable diets: Vegan, Vegetarian, Paleo
Servings: 2 (small-ish) smoothies

Calories*: 446 kcal
Protein*: 16.5 g
Carbs*: 32.7 g
Fat*: 31 g (26 grams of which saturates)
*Per portion

Ingredients:
- 1 ½ cups frozen mixed berries
- 1 cup coconut milk

- 2 tablespoons (naturally vegan) pea protein powder
- 1 tablespoon sweetener (such as honey, sugar, or agave syrup)
- 1 teaspoon raw cacao or cocoa powder
- 1 teaspoon sugar-free mixed berry jam or marmalade
- dark chocolate shavings

Instructions:

Add all the ingredients into a blender. (Tip: if you add the dry ingredients last, they tend to not stick to the bottom of the mixer.) Blend until smooth, and add more dark chocolate shavings to the top when serving.

If you're storing this smoothie in the fridge, it tends to thicken up due to the coconut milk. I recommend adding 1/3 cup water and mixing well if I know that I'll put it in the fridge overnight to take with me to work the next morning, for example.

Variations:

Chia seeds pack an extra punch of powerful protein. Remember that they absorb a lot of water, so if you add 1 tablespoon to the smoothie, it's best to add between ½ and 1 cup of water to the smoothie, depending on whether you'll consume it immediately or save in the fridge for later.

Spicy Cajun Mixed Nuts

Feel free to choose any type of nuts you'd like. So that they're easier to eat as finger food, I prefer using whole nuts rather than halved or chopped. Raw nuts also absorb the spicy oil mixture better than nuts that are already roasted.

Prep time: 5 min.
Cook time: 10 min.
Storage time: 7-10 days in an airtight container
Suitable diets: Vegan, Vegetarian, High Protein
Servings: 10 handful-sized portions

Nutritional information is largely dependent upon the types of nuts you choose to use. Therefore, I haven't included any here for this recipe. If you'd like me to amend this in future editions of the book, please say so in the comments on Amazon!

Ingredients:
- 5 ounces unsalted cashews
- 5 ounces shelled pecans
- 5 ounces shelled pistachios
- 1 tablespoon soft brown sugar (packed when measured*)
- 1 tablespoon olive oil
- 1 teaspoon smoked paprika
- 1 teaspoon powdered cayenne pepper
- 1 teaspoon finely ground Himalayan salt

- ½ teaspoon dried thyme
- ½ teaspoon black pepper, finely ground
- 1 baking sheet lined with wax parchment or 'baking paper'

Packing brown sugar down into the spoon or measuring cup makes a big difference in a recipe. Because more sugar is used when it's packed down, it can change the consistency of a recipe as well as the taste. I remember a story from my grandmother very vividly, as a reminder to always pack down brown sugar! My grandmother gave a tried-and-true recipe for banana bread to her friend. She used the recipe for many, many years and it's still a favorite in the family. This friend, however, had baked the recipe a few times and it always turned out 'wrong'; it didn't bake through the middle or it burned on the edges or it was just simply too dry and crumbly. My grandmother suddenly awoke at 3am, sitting upright in bed. "She's not packing the brown sugar!" she cried aloud. And it was true! Her friend made the changes to the measurements, and the recipe turned out perfectly.

Instructions:

Preheat the oven to 350°F or gas mark 4.

Combine the powdered ingredients and sugar in a small bowl, so they blend smoothly and evenly. Then, put all of the nuts into a large bowl. Sprinkle the powdered mixture into the nuts and stir well.

Then, add the olive oil and mix well. Pour out the nuts onto the wax baking paper, spreading them out so there are no clumps or clusters.

Bake for 5 minutes, stir the nuts, then bake for another 5 minutes. Let them cool completely before spooning into serving bowls or an airtight container.

Storage Tip: Save old pickle jars, olive jars, and other glass jars. After washing, let a mixture of bleach and water or vinegar and water sit in the jar overnight, to remove any odors from the jar's previous 'tenants'. Use these glass storage containers in lieu of plastic ones. Especially if you're storing food for more than a day, the 'taste' of plastic seeps into the food, distorting its flavor. There is already considerable research available testifying to the seepage of micro-plastic into our food, water, and environment in a very slow but steady pace. That causes a toxic build-up and a variety of health problems that I won't expound upon here. Check the appendix for further references and reading!

Protein-Packed Nachos

Nachos are a fun, easy, finger food the whole family can enjoy. Just like with pizza, if one member of the family doesn't like a certain ingredient, for example olives of jalapenos, then they can simply be sprinkled on the other side of the nacho tray before going in the oven.

Prep time: 15 min.
Bake time: 10 min.
Storage time: Half day before they get soggy
Suitable diets: Vegan, Vegetarian, Gluten-Free
Servings: 4-6 adult-sized portions

Because the portion size may vary, I haven't included nutritional information.

Ingredients:
- 2 cups pinto beans (also called black-eyes peas)
- 1 cup of kidney beans
- ½ cup jalapenos
- 1 large bag of tortilla chips (unsalted, if you can find any)
- 1 tablespoon olive oil or avocado oil
- ½ teaspoon ground cayenne pepper
- ½ teaspoon ground black pepper

- Himalaya salt
- 3 spring onions or scallions, thinly sliced
- 1 jar of guacamole OR two avocados smashed up with salt, pepper, and a teaspoon of oil
- 1 jar of salsa*
- Baking sheet lined with wax baking paper or baking parchment

If you prefer to make your own salsa, a simple recipe I use is: 4 chopped tomatoes, ½ white onion finely chopped, 2 tablespoons of olive oil, 1 tablespoon lime juice, and a sprinkle of white pepper and salt.

Instructions:

Preheat the oven to 350°F or gas mark 4.

Drain the water from the cans of beans. Alternatively you can get dried beans, soak them in water overnight, then boil in unsalted water for 30-40 minutes or until soft. To save time, I often used unsalted, no-frills, canned beans.

In a large bowl, combine the beans with oil, peppers and salt. Leave the jalapenos for sprinkling on last, in case some prefer to leave it off their portion of the nachos.

Spread out the tortilla chips on the baking sheet evenly. Place the beans mixture on top, sprinkling the spring onions and jalapenos on top. Bake for about 10 minutes.

Serve with salsa and guacamole on the side.

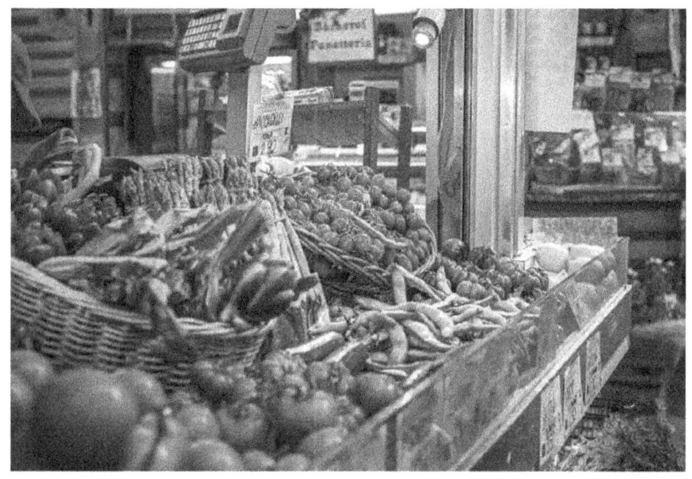

[5] Meal Plans, Shopping Lists & Real-Life Implementation

In this chapter I've included everything you need to help make trips to the grocery store easy on your wallet and give you maximum effect for the time you spend shopping. The next sections are divided into: helpful tips for shopping, meal plans for the week, and shopping lists so that you can buy one week's worth of food at once, and cook the meal plans as the week goes by.

I've devised these shopping lists and meal plans based upon a family of four (two adults, two children) but obviously feel free to cut the list quantities in half and cut the recipes in half. Alternatively, you can make some extra when you're cooking, to throw in the freezer if you are cooking for one – that is, only for yourself.

[5.1] Grocery Shopping Tips & Online Buying Guide

Generally, I do one big shopping trip every two weeks for the staples: toilet paper, paper towels, potatoes, grains, cereals, non-dairy milks, etc. and this is reflected in the shopping list section coming up later on in this chapter. You can also order this delivered – consolidating your trips to the store cuts down on Co2 emissions, and saves time.

Depending on where you live and what your transportation situation is like, you'll want to 'top up' on fresh produce every now and again. For me, I enjoy daily trips to the supermarket around the corner because I can push my toddler in his stroller which calms him down for his afternoon nap. It's also less busy mid-afternoon than it is after or before work.

If you drive to a grocery store and can only manage picking up fresh produce once a week, that's fine, too. Just be careful you don't let your produce spoil after a few days! (See the next subchapter "Storage" for tips.)

There are general rules of thumb to follow if you want to ensure a successful shopping trip. First and foremost is: Never grocery shop when you're hungry. You'll inevitably buy more than you need, and usually more snacks and unhealthy things.

Try to buy things you can use in more than one meal. That ensures you won't have half of a head of lettuce sitting in your fridge for a week without any plans to use it. And if that is the case – freeze it! You can always put frozen veggies into a soup later on.

Online Shopping Tips

Online shopping can actually be cheaper than going to brick and mortar stores if you're smart about how you do it. I usually google around for coupons first – and download any apps for brands or stores if they're available. For the 'right to market to you' with push notifications (before you uninstall the app), you'll often get money off certain items or, say, $10 off when you spend $50 or more.

Certain items can be cheaper and higher quality to buy online. Generally, wine and spirits are better purchased online and shipped to your house. Those companies can have some great prices because they can cut down on overhead expenses. That means they don't pay for more employees to work at a brick and mortar location that receives customers, they don't pay for electricity or security or rent in those places, either. Their products tend to be higher quality and their customer service is excellent because – unlike a store getting foot traffic – they rely heavily on reviews and ratings online to promote trust in their business and products.

Check out Groupon for take-away meal deals. And check your local area for food sharing initiatives. Many restaurants, grocery stores, and hotels give away food that's just reached its 'sell-by' date. In fact, it's against the law in France to throw away food; it must be given away or put into a food waste bin that goes to composting or creating bio-ethanol. I love that concept!

Another way to save money is by purchasing the store's own brand rather than large, name-brand cereals or other products. I haven't bought Kellogg's cereals in years just because of their price. If your children complain, then you'll just have to remain firm and they'll get used to it. You might want to try storing those items in a glass container (which is better than the plastic packaging anyway) so they only see the food and not the branding. Or, cut out the brand-name from the old cereal box and tape it onto the glass jar that you fill up with the no-name cereal. Your kids will be none the wiser!

One last piece of advice is on buying nutritional supplements. <u>Always</u> buy high-quality, trusted brands. Your body won't be able to absorb nutrients from supplements that are prepared improperly, because they nutritional content may have been damaged during processing or packaging. These won't harm your body as such, but you won't be getting the nutritional components you want and need if they are poorly made.

One label / company I know and trust 100% is DoTerra. They're ethical from top to bottom, paying farmers much faster than is customary in the industry, and much more fairly / generously. Here's their website: https://www.doterra.com/US/en

And if you're in the UK or EU, I highly recommend the liquid supplements from LaVita (https://www.lavita.de). Unfortunately their website is only in German, but you can find resellers of their product, and find it on Amazon as well. It's the only supplement I've taken where I feel it working, giving my body and energy boost about 10-15 minutes after drinking it.

[5.2] 7-Day Meal Plans

The way I've created these, one shopping list will cover a 7-day meal plan. Plans are categorized by men / women / children / older folks. Special 7-day meal plans are designed to help you reverse and/or prevent certain diseases or conditions.

Paleo-Friendly & Vegan

It is hard to be paleo and vegan, that's true. One of the Paleo staples is gelatine or bone broth. This meal plan can help you pack in raw, whole foods in a paleo way.

I've intentionally used the same recipes and suggestions in the meal plan below twice, sometimes in succession. This is because I'm assuming you're cooking for 2 (yourself and your partner), and so the serving size of 4 can be evenly divided. If cooking for a family of 4 or 5, feel free to double recipes and freeze them or store in the fridge.

Day of Week	Breakfast	Lunch	Snack 1	Dinner	Snack 2 (or Dessert)
Sunday	Italian tomatoes on gluten-free, raw onion bread	Sweet potato chili with quinoa (or substitute lentils)	Chia coconut granola-free bars	Cauliflower burgers on a bed of lettuce	Chocolate superfood balls
Monday	Chocolate berry smoothie (make more for tomorrow)	Flaxseed crackers with nut cheese, tomatoes & fresh basil	Spicy Cajun nuts	Peanut coconut curry	Ginger tonic
Tuesday	Chocolate berry smoothie	Vietnamese summer rolls with avocado on the side	Raw mixed nuts	Lemongrass pumpkin soup	Chia coconut pudding (soak chia seeds in coconut

					milk 20 minutes, add coconut flakes on top)
Wednesday	Vietnamese summer rolls with sliced bell pepper	Flaxseed crackers with mashed avocado lemon & cilantro	Chia coconut granola-free bars	Low-cal veggie soup	Raw blueberry chocolate torte
Thursday	Soy yogurt with chopped nuts & chia seeds	Low-cal veggie soup	Chocolate berry smoothie (make more for tomorrow)	Peanut coconut curry	Chia coconut pudding
Friday	Chocolate berry smoothie	Flaxseed crackers with chickpea-free falafel, cucumber and carrot sticks	Spicy cajun nuts	Protein packed nachos	Raw blueberry chocolate torte
Saturday	Avocado & tofu scramble	Stuffed mushrooms with almond green beans	Avocado (spoon it out of the skin directly)	Veghetti with pesto & a side salad	Chocolate superfood balls

High-Protein or "Men's Meal Plan"

This is good for those on the Atkins and Paleo diets, because the recipes in here are high in protein. They're also suitable for anyone working out and lifting weights.

Day of Week	Breakfast	Lunch	Snack 1	Dinner	Snack 2 (or Dessert)
Sunday	High protein chia oatmeal	Chickpea-free falafel with tofu salad	½ cup almonds	Sweet potato chili	Spicy cajun nuts
Monday	Avocado & tofu scramble	Pea soup with flaxseed crackers	½ cup almonds	Italian bean & barley stew	Chia coconut bars
Tuesday	Protein packed berry smoothie	Italian bean & barley stew	½ cup walnuts	Chili & rice stew	Cinnamon almond breakfast muffins
Wednesday	High protein chia oatmeal	Chickpea-free falafel with tofu salad	½ cup almonds	Sweet potato chili	Spicy cajun nuts
Thursday	Flaxseed crackers with nut cheese & avocado	Chili & rice stew	½ cup walnuts	Cashew salad	Cinnamon almond breakfast muffins
Friday	Avocado & tofu scramble	Italian bean & barley stew	½ cup almonds	Protein packed nachos	Chia coconut bars
Saturday	Cinnamon almond breakfast muffins (substitute half the almonds for protein powder)	Pea soup with flaxseed crackers	½ cup walnuts	Chickpea-free falafel with tofu salad	Chocolate blueberry tofu tarte

Weight Loss or "Women's Meal Plan"

I truly don't mean to come across as sexist, but it is a fact that the large majority of people in weight loss programs are women. This meal plan focuses on lighter foods and recipes that fill you up, but help you lose weight.

Day of Week	Breakfast	Lunch	Snack 1	Dinner	Snack 2 (or Dessert)
Sunday	Potato pancakes	Low-cal veggie soup	½ cup fresh dates	Mashed cauliflower with almond green beans	Ginger tonic
Monday	Golden oatmeal	Potato pancakes with slices of marinated tofu	½ cup dried apricots	Low-cal veggie soup	½ cup fresh dates
Tuesday	Breakfast potatoes	Chickpea-free falafel on salad	1 banana	Ratatouille on rice	Chia bars
Wednesday	Golden oatmeal	Sweet potato enchiladas	½ cup fresh dates	Moroccan lentil soup	Cinnamon almond breakfast muffins
Thursday	Berry smoothie	Moroccan lentil soup	½ cup dried apricots	Low-cal veggie soup	½ cup fresh dates
Friday	Chia bars	Low-cal veggie soup	Cinnamon almond breakfast muffins	Ratatouille on rice	Chia bars
Saturday	Cinnamon almond breakfast muffins	Sweet potato enchiladas	½ cup dried apricots	Stuffed mushrooms with almond green beans	½ cup fresh dates

Anti-Inflammatory (Helps Against Arthritis, Gout & More)

You likely already know the foods that contribute to gout flare-ups and inflammation in the body: cow's milk (and other dairy products), seafood like shrimp, lobster and oysters, as well as wheat products and refined white sugar. Increase your intake of ginger and cinnamon -- I even recommend taking ginger powder capsules twice daily.

Day of Week	Breakfast	Lunch	Snack 1	Dinner	Snack 2 (or Dessert)
Sunday	Apple cinnamon French toast	Vietnamese summer rolls with avocado tofu scramble	1 cup fresh blueberries	Sweet potato chili with quinoa	Blueberry torte
Monday	Cinnamon almond breakfast muffins	Veggie soup	Ginger tonic	Mashed cauliflower with garlic and almond beans	1 cup fresh blueberries
Tuesday	Breakfast potatoes	Sweet potato chili with quinoa	1 cup fresh blueberries	Veggie soup	Ginger tonic
Wednesday	Cinnamon almond breakfast muffins	Vietnamese summer rolls with avocado tofu scramble	Ginger tonic	Ratatouille with baked potatoes	1 cup fresh blueberries
Thursday	Apple cinnamon French toast	Lemongrass pumpkin soup (with extra ginger!)	1 cup fresh blueberries	Mashed cauliflower with garlic and almond beans	Ginger tonic
Friday	Soy yogurt with chopped nuts and dates	Protein smoothie with cinnamon, apple juice & collagen powder	Cinnamon almond breakfast muffins	Protein packed nachos	Blueberry torte
Saturday	Protein smoothie	Lemongrass pumpkin soup	Ginger tonic	Ratatouille on rice	Cinnamon almond

	with cinnamon, apple juice & collagen powder	(with extra ginger!)			breakfast muffins

Child-Friendly

This meal plan contains recipes that do not have much spice or 'weird' foods like mushrooms that children may not like the consistency or taste of.

Day of Week	Breakfast	Lunch	Snack 1	Dinner	Snack 2 (or Dessert)
Sunday	Apple cinnamon fresh toast	Lemongrass pumpkin soup	Flaxseed crackers with nut cheese	Ratatouille on rice	Cinnamon almond breakfast muffins
Monday	Avocado & tofu scramble	Spaghetti with red sauce	Flaxseed crackers with nut cheese	Lemongrass pumpkin soup	½ cup fresh grapes
Tuesday	Cinnamon almond breakfast muffins	P&J sandwich	fresh apple	Sweet potato enchiladas	Lemon pistachio cookies
Wednesday	Avocado & tofu scramble	Vietnamese summer rolls with veggie sticks	Flaxseed crackers with nut cheese	Ratatouille on rice	½ cup fresh grapes
Thursday	Cinnamon almond breakfast muffins	Sweet potato enchiladas	Flaxseed crackers with nut cheese	Veggie soup	½ cup fresh blueberries
Friday	Berry smoothie	Falafel on salad	½ cup fresh grapes	Protein packed nachos	Lemon pistachio cookies
Saturday	Potato pancakes	Vietnamese summer rolls with veggie sticks	Cinnamon almond breakfast muffins	Ratatouille on rice	½ cup fresh grapes

[5.3] Storage, Stocking, Freezing & Preparing

Planning and preparation are absolutely vital in a lifestyle shaped around healthy eating. If your veggies are going bad, cut off the black, wilted, or brown spots and cook the rest in a soup. Or if you don't have time to cook that day, throw them in the freezer until you can use them in a soup, stew, or baked casserole.

Here are some **tips for storing produce** to minimize or eliminate food waste:

1. Store lighter and softer produce gently so they don't bruise; For example, put kiwis, plums, tomatoes, pears, oranges and other soft fruits on the top of the produce crisper drawer in the fridge. Heavier things can be on the bottom, like most vegetables.

2. If you store a portion of the fruits and veggies you've bought in the fridge, that will extend their shelf life so they don't ripen (and then possibly over-ripen) too soon, before you can use them. I generally put out half in a bowl on the counter, and the other half in the fridge.

3. Never store produce in plastic bags! The produce can't 'breathe', condensation (water droplets) builds up, and produce spoils much faster – yes, even in the fridge. It's best to put **unwashed** produce into bags made of mesh, cloth, or brown paper.

4. Carrots and celery tend to wilt and 'pucker up' when out of their plastic packaging that they're sold in. I cut small slits on either end of their plastic packaging, and lay them slit-side down on top of a couple folded paper towels in the crisper drawer. This allows for the water droplet build-up to trickle out, but not let the carrots dry out.

5. Save time by preparing produce. I usually make time to prepare produce every 2-3 days. I call my family or friends to catch up and chop up lots of veggies at the same time. Bell peppers, carrots, celery, radishes, asparagus, brussels sprouts, cabbage, cauliflower, fennel, apples, mangoes and other 'firmer' produce store very well in glass jars filled with water. You can cover them or leave them uncovered. You don't need to add any Vitamin C (or lemon juice, which is

commonly used) to keep them from turning brown. They'll generally last 2-4 days in water staying crisp and firm, ready to use them when you need or to snack on easily.

6. Never store bananas in the fridge. They'll go brown more easily but just not ripen.

7. If you do have over-ripe or brown bananas, put them in the freezer until you can bake with them – it's actually better to bake with brown bananas, because they're sweeter and much easier to cream (mix with sugar and butter).

8. Tomatoes, lemons, limes, onions, garlic, and potatoes can be stored in the fridge but it's best to put them in a cool place away from direct sunlight. Same with mushrooms, as they tend to get slimy rather quickly at cooler fridge temperatures (which increase water condensation).

9. Store asparagus upright in a glass, mug, or glass jar with an inch or two of water at the bottom. This keeps them from drying up from the bottom up, becoming more brittle and chewy. This is especially the case for green asparagus which is the most common type sold in the states.

10.

Do you have any more tips or tricks for storing produce? I'd love to hear about them, and other readers would be grateful for the knowledge as well. Simply leave a comment on the Kindle book or on Amazon and let us know!

I'd like to reiterate a very helpful time-saving tip: Prepare sauces and side dishes when you have some time, for example a chilled-out Saturday night watching Netflix as you shell garbanzo beans. Or making sauces as you chat on the phone with family. You can prepare sauces, chop vegetables for the next few days, and do other preparation that will save you time when your busy week starts.

Manage your time well. If you're chopping up onions, maybe do the whole bag and freeze half. Consider buying one of those veggie choppers to make it go faster – they're either electric or manual, and you can find them on Amazon for as little as $10 – or even less if you find it on Facebook Marketplace from a neighbor, or at a garage sale nearby.

[5.4] Foods to Completely Avoid

In general, avoid any pre-packaged 'ready meals' or packaged foods such as:

1. Frozen ready meals (they're often high in sodium and refined sugar)
2. Packaged food that contains high fructose corn syrup
3. Chips, Doritos, Pringles, and the like – they have too much oil and salt
4. Cookies, pastries, cakes, or other sugary desserts – you can make your own that are healthier, without the chemicals, additives, dyes, and white sugar
5. Bread, grains, and cereals if you're on a Paleo diet. (See Chapter 3 for more details.)
6. Meat, red meat, poultry, and fish – if you're serious about being plant-based, then you'll eliminate beef, pork, lamb, fish, seafood, and the like.
7. Honey, eggs, cow/goat/sheep's milk and other dairy like butter made from animal sources – this would constitute a vegan as well as plant-based diet

[5.5] How to Deal with Cravings

Getting off of refined sugar is like coming off drugs. It can create serious withdrawal symptoms that affect your mood, behavior, energy levels and even hormones – ever notice how eating too much sugar often makes you break out with acne? That doesn't happen because sugar is oily, but because it affects your hormonal system and your body's way of processing sugar, oils, and carbohydrates – essentially the fuels your body uses as energy.

Gradually transition yourself off sugar by cutting down on the amount you consume every day. Take it slow, and do this at a time when you don't have much stress in other areas of your life.

Eat plenty of dried fruits (ones without sugar added, such as apricots or apple chips) to satisfy your sweet tooth, and top up with stevia, coconut blossom syrup, maple syrup, xylitol or other natural sweeteners. It's true, they don't taste exactly like sugar – but don't focus on what you're *not* getting. Focus on enjoying the food you have. Your sugar cravings will be quite strong within the 3 days you start coming off it. After about 2-3 weeks you won't have any cravings anymore. I can promise you that you'll have less 'brain fog' and enjoy more of a steady calm demeanor throughout the day rather than the highs and lows (especially after lunchtime).

One product I absolutely love is developed by a ground-breaking company in California. I don't have time to fully explore the microbiome and gut health in this book, but you can find more information on their website about how they create a 'microbial soup' of bacteria and other cultures that are good for our gut. They then put this good mixture into harmful substances like chocolate, coffee, and sugar. Placing a bit of this substance under your tongue and holding it there for about a minute helps 'reset' your brain as well as your gut. You'll find that your taste buds recognize the harmful substance (like sugar), but the fermentation with good bacteria is also picked up by your body as a positive signal, as a substance your body wants more than the sugar. Find more information on their website https://biometech.com/.

[5.6] Setting Up Strong Habits for Your Health

Don't expect to suddenly change your entire life around overnight. Many people find success making gradual changes rather than 'going cold turkey'. Here are some tips:

- Use food tracking or calorie counting apps like MyFitnessPal
- Use the paper version: writing meals and snacks in a journal
- Write down your goals for the week, 3 weeks, and 6 weeks to remind yourself of where you want to be — maybe it's realistic, maybe you'll have to amend as you go along
- Keep a journal of your feelings, mood, and quality of sleep — I can guarantee you'll feel better and better as you eat healthier
- Set milestones for motivation: working toward a goal of reducing / eliminating sugar, reaching a certain weight or

body measurement, fitting into a cute outfit or pair of jeans again

- If you're looking to lose weight, measure yourself! Muscle weighs more than fat, so you'll notice changes in how your clothes feel (i.e. shedding inches before pounds) before you notice much difference on the scale.
- Get a meal plan buddy: a family member, neighbor, friend or someone on a FB group or forum to share recipes, inspire, motivate, and hold each other accountable.
- Write yourself 'love notes', encouraging affirmations taped up around your home and office
- Listen to podcasts, read blogs, watch documentaries and surround yourself with people who are positive and informational about the topic of plant-based diets. You'll learn more and motivate yourself to continue.

[5.7] Shopping Lists

Many of the recipes use largely the same ingredients -- that was intentional, so you can make 2-3 recipes from the same ingredients, which eliminates food waste.

List 1

- PRODUCE
- 1 bag of sweet potatoes (usually 5-8 in a bag)
- 1 large bag of white potatoes (usually 2 pounds)
- 1 bag of white or yellow onions (usually 1 pound, about 5-6 onions)
- 1 large pumpkin
- 1 medium butternut squash
- 1 head of lettuce
- 1 bag of carrots (usually 2 pounds)
- 1 bag of celery (usually about 1 pound)
- 1 bag of apples
- frozen blueberries
- fresh blueberries (optional)

- 1 bag of 3-5 fresh lemons

- OTHER AISLES
- 1 package of oats (not instant)
- 1 package of barley
- 1 bottle of extra virgin olive oil
- cashews
- almonds
- almond or soy milk (optional)

- SUGARS & SPICES
- xylitol
- stevia (usually comes powdered in a jar)
- honey (optional - if you're not vegan)
- coconut blossom or agave syrup
- ground cinnamon
- ground ginger
- lemongrass (whole and fresh, sold in packages of 5-6)
- fresh ginger (about the size of your hand… if you have extra you don't use for cooking, simply make ginger tea with lemon)

List 2

- PRODUCE
- 1 bag of sweet potatoes (usually 5-8 in a bag)
- 1 large bag of white potatoes (usually 2 pounds)
- 1 bag of white or yellow onions (usually 1 pound, about 5-6 onions)
- 1 head of lettuce
- 1 bag of carrots (usually 2 pounds)
- 3-5 bell peppers
- 2 zucchinis
- 1 eggplant
- 4-5 avocados
- 1 bag of apples

- 1 bag of 3-5 fresh lemons
- 1-2 fresh limes (or a bottle of lime juice)
- other fruits: bananas, oranges, others for snacking like fresh dates

- OTHER AISLES
- 1 package of oats (not instant)
- 1 package of barley
- 1 package of rice
- 2-3 packages of dried beans (kidney, pinto, black-eyed, butter)
- 1 bottle of extra virgin olive oil
- cashews
- almonds
- almond or soy milk (optional)
- 2 blocks of tofu, firm (or smoked)

- SUGARS & SPICES
- xylitol
- stevia (usually comes powdered in a jar)
- honey (optional - if you're not vegan)
- coconut blossom or agave syrup
- ground cinnamon
- ground ginger
- lemongrass (whole and fresh, sold in packages of 5-6)
- chili flakes or fresh chilis
- smoked paprika

[Appendix]

[A] Conversions of Measurements and Temperatures

Liquid Measurements

United States / Australia	United Kingdom ("Imperial")	Metric
	1 fluid ounce (= fl oz)	25ml
¼ cup	2 fl oz	60ml
	3 fl oz	75ml
	3 ½ fl oz	100ml
½ cup	4 fl oz	120ml
	5 fl oz	150ml
¾ cup	6 fl oz	180ml
	7 fl oz	200ml
1 cup	9 fl oz	250ml
1.25 cups	10 ½ fl oz	300ml
1.5 cups	12 ½ fl oz	350ml
1.75 cups	14 fl oz	400ml
2 cups	16 fl oz	450ml
2.5 cups	1 pint	600ml
3 cups	1 ¼ pints	750ml (bottle of wine size)
4 cups or 1 quart	1 ¾ pints	1000ml or 1 liter

| 1.5 quarts | 2 ¾ pints | 1.5 liters |
| 2 quarts | 3 ½ pints | 2 liters |

Solid / "Dry" Measurements

These are, for example, all-purpose flour and oats. Sugar is considered a 'wet' ingredient because it can actually 'dry out' after months of sitting in the pantry. Brown sugar is typically packed (squashed down into the measuring cup) unless otherwise stated in the recipe. Brown sugar is the heaviest of all; ½ cup of packed brown sugar weighs 110 grams or nearly 4 ounces!

1/8 cup (or 2 tablespoons)	16 grams	0.536 ounces
¼ cup	32 g	1.13 oz
1/3 cup	43 g	1.5 oz
½ cup	64 g	2.25 oz
⅔ cup	85 g	3 oz
¾ cup	96 g	3.38 oz
1 cup	128 g	4.5 oz

Oven Temperature Conversions

	Celcius (°C)	Fahrenheit (°F)	Gas Mark
Very cool – best used for keeping pancakes or French Toast warm while cooking the rest	110-120	225-250	¼ – ½
Cool – best for reheating leftovers	140-150	275-300	1-2
Medium – some casseroles and other dishes that may burn easily	160-170	325-350	3-4
Medium Hot – most cakes, muffins and "breads" like banana bread are baked between medium and medium hot	190-200	375-400	5-6
Hot – Braising and 'crisping' potatoes or other legumes on their edges for a nice, crunchy effect	220-230	425-450	7-8
Very Hot – crème brulée with cow's milk or other dairy is often baked very hot. The plant-based alternatives we use here would scorch and be ruined at this temperature!	240	475	9

[B] Quick Reference: Food Replacements & Substitutes

These have been discussed in more detail in the book, and have been compiled here for your convenience as a quick reference.

Vegan

1 egg = 1 medium-sized banana

cheese = raw nut cheese (see our recipe above)

1 cup honey = ⅔ cup stevia or xylitol

1 cup cow milk = 1 cup soy / almond / nut milk (be careful of the consistency, that whatever you're baking doesn't become too 'chewy' with this non-dairy milk -- that's why I usually add baking soda and vinegar to my baking recipes, to get that fluffy light texture)

Higher Protein

If using flour for baking or cooking, substitute half that amount with almond meal (ground up almonds) or other nuts.

Slip in another scoop of protein powder into a soup or recipe…. you may need to add 2 tablespoons of water to compensate for the extra dryness.

Where you can, substitute nuts for carbohydrates (like chips or rice). Remember, this will have a higher fat and calorie count.

Low Sugar & Low Salt

Salt: Try to use Himalayan 'Pink' salt when you can, because it naturally has a higher amount of minerals than iodized table salt. If the recipe allows, use soy sauce or Bragg's Amino Acids instead (it tastes just like soy sauce). They have lower sodium levels and more nutrition. You might not want to substitute Bragg's Amino Acids for salt in a recipe for cupcakes, for example, but perhaps in savory breakfast muffins, soup, or casseroles.

Proper Food Combining

Replace fruits with sweet-tasting vegetables.

- Apple, baked = Sweet potato, baked
- Cheese = Vegan cheese or oil
- Cream = Soy cream or other alternative to dairy; in a pinch, throw soft tofu in a blender with one small white potato or one cup steamed cauliflower to maintain a 'creamy' consistency
- Oranges, baked or glazed = Carrots or sweet potatoes, baked or glazed
- Raspberries, jellied or jammed = Sunflower (or other) seeds with lemon or ascorbic acid (Vitamin C) for the sour or tangy flavor

[C] Rules for Proper Food Combining

1. Only eat fruit alone, on an empty stomach. It's best to do this first thing in the morning, otherwise wait 4 hours for your stomach to completely empty its contents.

2. Don't combine protein and grains. This means meat, fish, nuts, beans, and seeds (which are proteins) shouldn't be combined with rice, pasta, bread, potatoes, or other grains.

3. It's okay to combine grains with vegetables OR proteins with vegetables.

4. Don't drink more than 4 ounces half an hour before a meal, during a meal, or up to 2 hours after a meal.

[D]   References   and   Helpful Resources for Further Reading

The following books, articles, and people have greatly helped me in writing this book. They're worth taking a look at for further inspiration! (And for anyone reading this outside the USA, I've included only the US ISBNs for reference. They may differ in your country.)

- <u>Dick Gregory's Natural Diet for Folks Who Eat</u>. Dick Gregory. 1974 by Harper & Row Publishing House.
- <u>Easy Vegan: Simple Recipes for Healthy Eating</u>. Publishing Director: Alison Starling. First published in 2010 by Ryland Peters & Small. ISBN: 978 1 84597 958 4.
- <u>Eat Drink Paleo: Over 110 Paleo-Inspired Recipes for Everyone</u>. Irena Macri. Published by Penguin Random House in 2015. ISBN: 978 0 718 18165 9.
- <u>First-Time Vegan: Delicious Dishes and Simple Switches for a Plant-Based Lifestyle</u>. Leah Vanderveldt. Published in 2019 by Ryland Peters & Small. ISBN: 978 1 78879 062 8.
- <u>Fresh Vegan Kitchen: Delicious Recipes for the Vegan & Raw Kitchen</u>. David and Charlotte Bailey. First published in 2018 by Pavilion. UK ISBN: 978 1 911624 07 3.
- <u>Gino's Veg Italia! The Healthier Way to Eat Italian</u>. Gino D'Acampo. Published by Hodder & Stoughton in 2015. eBook ISBN: 978 1 444 79520 2.
- <u>Natural Health, Sugar and the Criminal Mind</u>. J. I. Rodale. 1968. Published by Pyramid Books of New York.
- <u>The Encyclopedia of Healing Foods</u>. Micheal Murray, Joseph Pizzorno, Lara Pizzorno. Published by Atria Books in 2005. ISBN: 978 0 7434 7402 3.
- <u>The Encyclopedia of Natural Medicine</u>. Micheal Murray, Joseph Pizzorno. Published by Prima Publishing in California. ISBN: 0 7615 1157 1.
- <u>The Gluten-Free Cookbook</u>. Heather Whinney and Fiona Hunter. Published by
- Dorling Kindersley Ltd in 2015. ISBN: 9780241185674.

- <u>The Paleo Primer: A Second Helping</u>. Keris Marsden and Matt Whitmore. Published by Watkins Media Limited 2017. ISBN: 978 1 84899 341 9.
- <u>The Raw Food Diet: The Healthy Way to Get the Shape You Want</u>. Christine Bailey. Published by Duncan Baird in 2012. ISBN: 978 1 84483 994 0.
- <u>The Uncook Book: The Essential Guide to a Raw Food Lifestyle</u>. Tanya Maher. Published by Hay House Inc. in 2015. ISBN: 978 1 78180 564 0.
- <u>Without the Calories, Quick and Easy: Losing Weight Is As Easy As 1-2-3</u>. Justine Pattison. Published by Orion Books in 2018. UK ISBN: 978 1 4091 5471 6 (referenced for imperial measurement conversions, hence the UK number).
- <u>Vegetables</u>. Antonio Carluccio. First published in 2016 by Quadrille Publishing. ISBN: 978 184949 752 7.

Acknowledgements

I'm very thankful to my supportive family for the help and encouragement they've given me along the way. This wouldn't be possible without them!

I'm also very grateful to Kasey Phifer of The Bristol Centre for Biofeedback for her advice and input regarding the nutrients, gut health, and other valuable insights into the human digestive tract.

I'm also very thankful to Harvey and Marilyn Diamond for their book "Food For Life" which introduced my family and me to proper food combining. Their rules (or whomever invented them) have been adapted in this book.

About the Author

Silvia Pala is Italian, and after travelling extensively she's settled down in Italy with her husband Marco and two children. She currently manages a translation and copywriting company while enjoying nature and good food with family on the weekends.

Download my FREE booklet: *Plant-based Diet for Beginners: 10 Simple & Healthy Plant-based Recipes Ready in 10 Minutes or Less*
URL: https://forms.aweber.com/form/70/510894270.htm

Amazon Author Page
URL: https://www.amazon.com/Silvia-Pala/e/B081F8SBBW/

Newsletter - Receive 10 FREE Best Plant-Based Recipes – a new one for 10 days – starting from TODAY
URL: https://forms.aweber.com/form/59/1338605359.htm

FB Group:
Please join my Facebook group to receive the latest updates, recipes, news and much more on plant-based diets
URL: https://www.facebook.com/groups/121951289126430/